DISORDERED DEFAECATION

DEVELOPMENTS IN SURGERY

J.M. Greep, H.A.J. Lemmens, D.B. Roos, H.C. Urschel (eds.), Pain in Shoulder and Arm: An Integrated View. 1979. ISBN 90 247 2146 6

B. Niederle, Surgery of the Biliary Tract. 1981. ISBN 90 247 2402 3

J.A. Nakhosteen & W. Maassen (eds.), Bronchology: Research, Diagnostic and Therapeutic Aspects. 1981. ISBN 90 247 2449 X

R. van Schilfgaarde, J.C. Stanley, P. van Brummelen & E.H. Overbosch (eds.), Clinical Aspects of Renovascular Hypertension. 1983. ISBN 0 89838 574 1

G.M. Abouna (ed.) & A.G. White (ass. ed.), Current Status of Clinical Organ Transplantation. With some Recent Developments in Renal Surgery. 1984. ISBN 0 89838 635 7

A. Cuschieri & G. Berci, Common Bile Duct Exploration. 1984. ISBN 0 89838 639 X

F.M.J. Debruyne & Ph.E.V.A. van Kerrebroeck, Practical Aspects of Urinary Incontinence. 1986. ISBN 0 89838 752 3

H.G. Gooszen, H.O. ten Cate Hoedemaker, I.T. Weterman & M.R.B. Keighley (eds.), Disordered Defaecation. 1987. ISBN 0 89838 891 0

S. Bengmark (ed.), Progress in Surgery of the Liver, Pancreas and Biliary System. 1987. ISBN 0 89838 956 9

DISORDERED DEFAECATION

Current opinion on diagnosis and treatment

edited by

H.G. GOOSZEN and H.O. TEN CATE HOEDEMAKER
Department of Surgery, University Hospital
Leiden, The Netherlands

I.T. WETERMAN
Department of Gastroenterology, University Hospital
Leiden, The Netherlands

M.R.B. KEIGHLEY
Department of Surgery, The General Hospital
Birmingham, United Kingdom

1987 **MARTINUS NIJHOFF PUBLISHERS**
a member of the KLUWER ACADEMIC PUBLISHERS GROUP
DORDRECHT / BOSTON / LANCASTER

Distributors

for the United States and Canada: Kluwer Academic Publishers, P.O. Box 358, Accord Station, Hingham, MA 02018-0358, USA
for the UK and Ireland: Kluwer Academic Publishers, MTP Press Limited, Falcon House, Queen Square, Lancaster LA1 1RN, UK
for all other countries: Kluwer Academic Publishers Group, Distribution Center, P.O. Box 322, 3300 AH Dordrecht, The Netherlands

Library of Congress Cataloging in Publication Data

```
Disordered defaecation.

   (Developments in surgery)
   Based on a Boerhaave course organized by the Faculty
of Medicine, University of Leiden, The Netherlands.
   Includes bibliographies and index.
   1. Defecation disorders--Congresses.  I. Gooszen, H. G.
II. Rijksuniversiteit te Leiden.  Faculteit der
Geneeskunde.  III. Series.  [DNLM: 1. Anus Diseases--
physiopathology.  2. Defecation.  3. Rectal Diseases--
physiopathology.  W1 DE998S / WI 600 D612]
RC866.D43D57  1987      616.3'5        87-11095
```

ISBN-13: 978-94-010-7998-3   e-ISBN-13: 978-94-009-3335-4
DOI: 10.1007/978-94-009-3335-4

Copyright

Contents

Contents

VI

3.   FAECAL INCONTINENCE

Preface

This book is a unique work devoted to the subject of disordered defaecation. It contains chapters written by experts in the field of ano-rectal physiology and management of disordered defaecation. The various contributions present personal views and special clinical experience of individuals.

There are some personal views which we felt should be commented upon and a few areas where the experience of others has been included into the text. For the sake of completeness of each chapter, a slight overlap in some cases was inevitable.

We hope the book will serve as a useful collection of opinions on a subject which until recently has been largely ignored by the medical profession.

The editors

Major contributors

H.O. ten Cate Hoedemaker
Department of Surgery, University Hospital, Rijnsburgerweg 10, 2333 AA Leiden, The Netherlands

G. Coremans
Department of Internal Medicine, University Hospital Gasthuisberg, Herestraat 49, 3000 Leuven, Belgium

S. Fasth
Department of Surgery II, Sahlgrenska Hospital, S-413 45 Göteborg, Sweden

H.G. Gooszen
Department of Surgery, University Hospital, Rijnsburgerweg 10, 2333 AA Leiden, The Netherlands

J.A. Gruwez
Department of General Surgery, University Hospitals KU, Brusselsestraat 63, 3000 Leuven, Belgium

M.M. Henry
Department of Gastroenterology, Central Middlesex Hospital, Acton Lane, London NW10 7NS, United Kingdom

M.R.B. Keighley
Department of Surgery, The General Hospital, Steelhouse Lane, Birmingham B4 6NH, United Kingdom

J.H.C. Kuypers
Department of Surgery, University Hospital St. Radboud, Geert Grooteplein Zuid 14, 6500 HB Nijmegen, The Netherlands

Ph.B. Miner
Division of Gastroenterology, Department of Medicine, University of Kan-

sas Medical Center, 39th and Rainbow Blvd., Kansas City, KS 66103, U.S.A.

N.J. McC Mortensen
Department of Surgery, Bristol Royal Infirmary, Bristol BS2 8HW, United Kingdom

R.J. Nicholls
Department of Surgery, St. Marks Hospital, City Road London EC1V 2PS, United Kingdom

N.W. Read
Subdepartment of Human Gastro-intestinal Physiology and Nutrition, Floor K, Royal Hallamshire Hospital, Glossop Road, Sheffield S10 2JF, United Kingdom

W.R. Schouten
Department of Surgery, University Hospital Dijkzigt, Dr. Molewaterplein 40, 3015 GD Rotterdam, The Netherlands

A.J.P.M. Smout
Department of Internal Medicine, University Hospital, Catharijnesingel 101, 3511 GV Utrecht, The Netherlands

S.J. Snooks
Department of Surgery, St. Bartholomew's Hospital, West Smithfield, London EC1A 7BE, United Kingdom

M. Swash
Department of Neurology, The London Hospital, Whitechapel, London E1 BB, United Kingdom

I.T. Weterman
Department of Gastroenterology, University Hospital, Rijnsburgerweg 10, 2333 AA Leiden, The Netherlands

N.S. Williams
Surgical Unit, The London Hospital, Whitechapel, London E1 BB, United Kingdom

N.R. Womack
Surgical Unit, The London Hospital, Whitechapel, London E1 BB, United Kingdom

1. Physiology

1.1 Anal and rectal manometry

H.O. TEN CATE HOEDEMAKER & H.G. GOOSZEN

Introduction

Ano-rectal manometry was first described by Gowers in 1877 [1]. In his initial report he focused on resting tone and recto-anal inhibitory reflex on filling of the rectum. With the introduction of more sophisticated technology into manometry apparently more detailed and more valuable information was obtained. Manometry, by measurement of pressure, supplies information about muscle activity at the time of actual measurement. Muscle activity gives relatively little information on the dynamics of muscle function and therefore supplies only limited information on the quality of muscle function in relation to the expected activity. The pressure measured in the anal canal at the level of the anal sphincters always has to be interpreted against the background of other factors playing a role in the function of the ano-rectum. Experience gained in manometry of the oesophagus and the lower oesophageal sphincter has demonstrated that considerable variation in pressures are registered on 24 hour manometry [2]. It is likely that fluctuations in pressure also occur at the level of the anal sphincters, since the sphincter mechanism shows different degrees of activity during the day. These considerations do, however, put into perspective the relative value of the data that are obtained with ano-rectal manometry.

When embarking on ano-rectal manometry in patients with all sorts of disorders of defaecation, it is important to gain insight in what sort of information manometry is supplying in relation to the equipment used.

In the next paragraphs the indications for ano-rectal manometry and the characteristics of the equipments currently available will be discussed.

The pressure profile

Using most common forms of manometry, intra-anal pressure is a low frequency signal showing a slow-wave pattern with a frequency of 10–20 waves per minute [1–3]. This is usually referred to as the 'basal sphincter pressure'. At sudden rises in intra-abdominal pressure, a high frequency signal is superimposed on the low frequency baseline pressure, the 'squeeze pressure'. The amplitude of these signals is determined by several factors and amongst these, the filling condition of the rectum [4].

The intra-anal pressure will show considerable variations during the day and overnight. These variations will, in normal controls, be determined by the presence or absence of faeces in the rectal ampulla, and posture. The most appropriate site for recording these pressures is hard to localize, since the anal canal is asymmetrical, the muscles contributing to intra-anal pressure are under different pathways of neural control and the influence of the anal wall itself is difficult to assess. At the cranial part of the anal canal, pressure is highest at the dorsal side, probable as a result of the puborectalis muscle which is fixed anteriorly to the pubis thus creating a loop around the rectum posteriorly. In the mid-anal canal, pressure is equally distributed over all quadrants, and in the lower anal canal pressure is highest anteriorly [5, 6].

The ano-rectal manometry equipment

Many sensors and transducers are currently available for measuring ano-rectal pressure. Equipment used for anal manometry is not always appropriate to study rectal manometry and therefore these fields of application will be discussed separately.

Anal manometry

Properties of the anal manometry equipment

In order to give optimal information on anal pressure profile the sensor and transducer must fulfil the following qualifications:
– the sensor must be as small as possible. It has been well documented that the pressure in the canal is influenced by the probe diameter [7, 8, 9] and the bigger the probe, the higher the resting tone: the sphincter stretching induced by a wide probe increases resting tone, the probe may be responsible for sphincteric contraction and contraction is more forceful with an increase in diameter.
– the transducer should be capable of picking up pressure signals with an amplitude ranging from 0 to at least 30 kPa. Studies by others [3, 7] have shown that intra-anal pressure ranges from 0 to 30 kPa as studied in normal

controls and in patients with intra-anal disease with documented elevation in resting intra-anal pressure amongst some patients with haemorrhoids and anal fissure [10, 11]. The transducer should however be capable of recording pressures upto 150 kPa, in order to sustain the high pressures that are applied in flushing procedures.

The electric signal changes must be proportional to the differences in pressure that occur in the anal canal. A deviation of 1% in the range 0–10 kPa is acceptable. This means a deviation of no more than 1 cm water pressure in measuring resting pressure.

- the sensitivity drift of the transducer should not exceed 0.1%/C. The change of the electrical output signal in reaction to the change in the pressure applied, is called the sensitivity of the transducer. One must notify that sensitivity changes with temperature[12]. Baseline drift up to 0.1 cm H_2O/C is acceptable. A transducer is usually calibrated at room temperature. After introduction into the anal, the temperature will rise by about 17° C. This means that because of the sensitivity drift a deviation of 1 to 2 cm water pressure may result. Thus in normal practice, a sensitivity drift of 1 to 2 cm H_2O pressure has to be accepted.

- The frequency response of the transducer must be at least 15 Hz. This means that a transducer must be capable of detecting a pressure change with an undistorted frequency of 15 cm H_2O. Almost all transducers currently in use for anal manometry fulfil this characteristic. The catheter connection to the transducer represents another possible limiting factor in frequency response. (see: Catheters).

The sensor is the indispensable part of the manometry equipment whereas pressure can be measured with or without a transducer.

Manometry equipment without a transducer

Transducers were not used in the early days of anal manometry. Figure 1 shows an example of such an apparatus with an intra-anal catheter directly connected to a water-infusion system. Only minimal baseline pressure can be measured and no information on squeeze pressure can be obtained, because water will leak into the anus, until the pressure level in the water column equals the lowest pressure in the anal canal. Furthermore, sphincteric contraction leads to occlusion of the sideholes. The method is elaborate because the water column has to be refilled at every study. The flow of water precipitates a sphincteric response and therefore interferes with a reliable recording of resting pressure. Figure 2 shows another example of manometry without a transducer [13]. An open-air perfused catheter is connected to a mercury blood pressure device. Air is inflated through the catheter into the anal canal. Pressure accumulates in the system until it exceeds the intra-anal pressure. Air

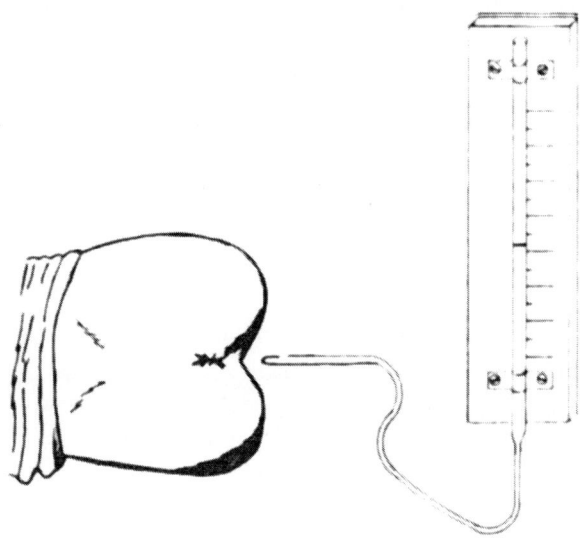

Figure 1. Water-perfused system.

will then escape from the anus. Although such a device is easy to be used and can provide basal and squeeze pressure data, no graphical representation of pressure/time-data can be obtained. Manometry equipment without a transducer no longer has a place in the investigation of ano-rectal function today.

Manometry equipment with transducer

The transducer can be in direct contact with the wall of the anal canal, but in most popular devices, there is a medium between the transducer and the anal wall.

Intra-anal transducers
Force gauge assembly catheter. A force gauge assembly catheter [5] (Figure 3) consists of a semi-rigid core with one or more force gauges attached to it. The strain gauge is part of an electrical circuit being one arm of a Wheatstone bridge. It is very expensive and the catheter is very fragile. With the introduction of the microtransducers, the use of this equipment has almost completely been abandoned.

Microtransducer catheter. A microtransducer (Figure 4) is mounted on a catheter [10, 14, 15, 16]. The size of the transducer varies but usually has a diameter of about 2 mm. The catheter has a lumen to provide a reference

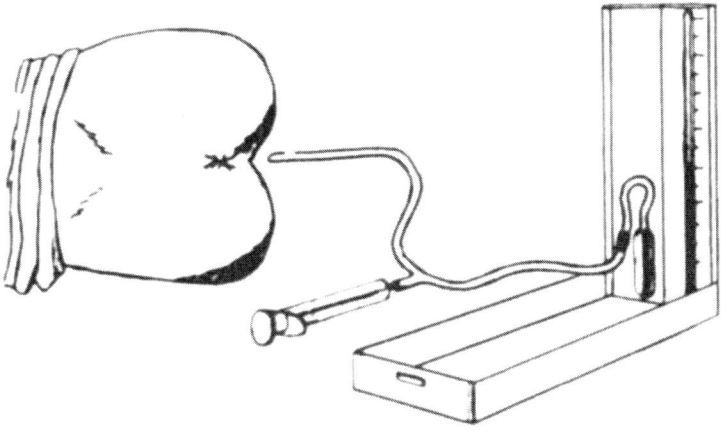

Figure 2. Air-perfused system with mercury column.

pressure (atmospheric pressure). The microtransducer is connected through fragile threads to the amplifier. These catheters are easy to handle, very stable (no baseline drift), because of their small size there is no increase in basal sphincter tone, but some catheters are too rigid. The relatively high cost, especially when a multisensor catheter is needed, is of course a disadvantage.

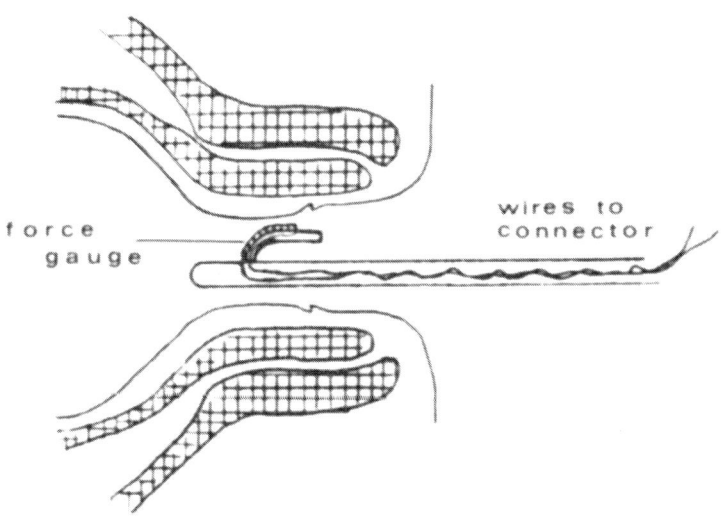

Figure 3. Force gauge assembly catheter.

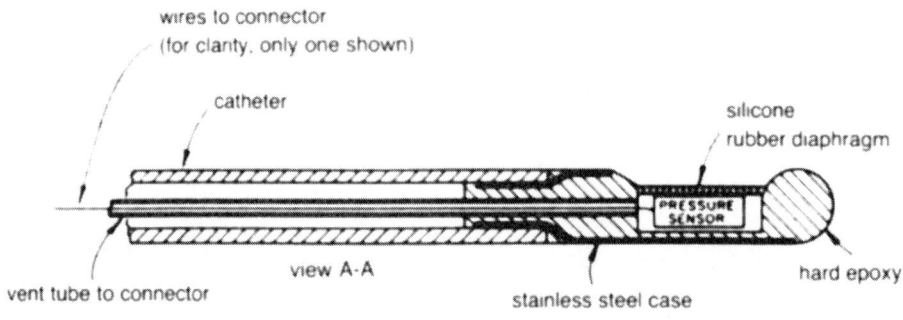

Figure 4. Microtransducer. (Baeten CGMI. Haemorrhoids, evaluation of methods of treatment. 1985. Thesis. Maastricht.)

Extra-anal transducers
With the transducer outside the anus, intra-anal pressure changes have to be transmitted to the transducer. An open or a closed system can be used for transmission, using air or fluid as the medium.

Closed systems
Air filled catheters. With these catheters, pressure waves are damped, because of the compressibility of air. Therefore the frequency response is poor, and a noncompressible medium such as water is more advisable.

Water filled catheters. Pressure waves are very accurately transported by water. A water filled catheter is most often used in connection with a balloon catheter. With an increase in balloon diameter the intra-anal resting pressure rises [3]. Another disadvantage is that balloon catheters show a considerable baseline drift, due to gradual change in balloon compliance [17]. For this reason the system has to be calibrated before and after measurement, which makes it elaborate. Balloon catheters can not detect directional change, only circumferential pressure.

Open systems
Open non-perfused catheters were used initially, but are inaccurate in col-

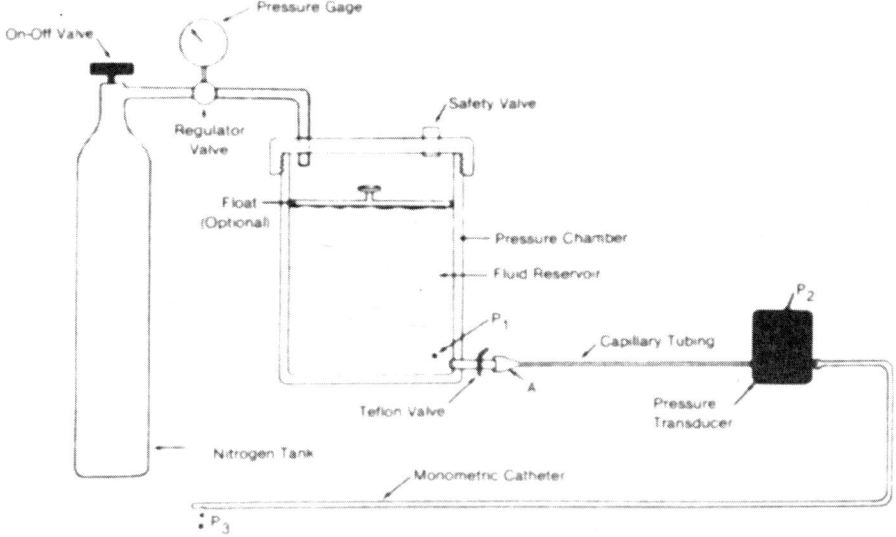

Figure 5. Low compliance pump. (Arndorfer RC, Stef JJ, Dodds WJ, Linehan JH, Hogan WJ. Improved infusion system for intraluminal esophageal manometry. Gastroenterology 1977; 73: 23–7)

lapsed organs, due to mucosa sealing off the catheter recording orifices [18]. This problem can be overcome by using water-perfused catheters. A modern infusion system consists of a low compliance pump according to Arndorfer (Figure 5) [18]. When the catheter orifice is not occluded by the anal mucosa, the system will record low pressures since the system will be at a level equal to the pressure at the tip of the catheter. When the anal canal mucosa presses against the orifice of the catheter, flow in the catheter will cease until the pressure in the system exceeds the anal wall pressure where upon flow will restart and an equilibrium will be attained at a pressure equal to the intra-anal pressure. Several factors influencing the frequency response of the system: the type of infusion pump, flow rate, catheter bore, orifice, length and compliance.

Syringe pump or high compliance pump (Figure 6). This type of pump [7, 19] is widely used. This type of pump must produce a rapid infusion rate of 6 cc per minute [19], in order to register intra-anal pressure fluctuations adequately. The system is relatively slow (Figure 7), because of its large compliance caused by the bigger volume. When the catheter is occluded at the tip, the pressure in the whole system will rise. This pressure rise is caused by movement of the piston. However, a substantial part of the pressure rise is lost because of the

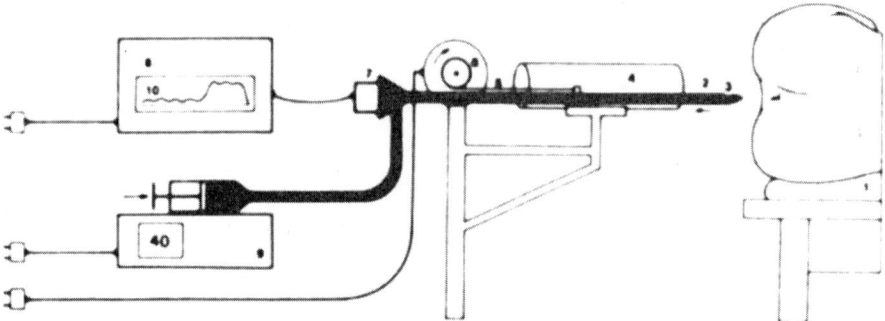

Figure 6. High compliance pump. (Kuypers JHC. Over de perianale fistel. 1981. Thesis. Nijmegen)

flexibility of the syringe, the syringe tends to increase in size. Owing to the compliance of the syringe an infusion rate of 6 ml per minute is required; unfortunately, this high flow rate easily causes a sphincteric response. This problem is even bigger with a multilumen catheter.

Normal values of intra-anal pressure

The basal or resting tone in the anal canal is the result of the combined activity of the internal and the external anal sphincter. Elevation of sphincter tone above the basal tone is the result of an increase in activity of the external anal sphincter. The contribution of the internal sphincter to the basal sphincter tone is estimated to amount to between 74% [20] and 85% [21] of the pressure measured. Others [22] state that the external sphincter only adds to the basal tone when a faecal bolus reaches the anal canal, which means that basal tone is almost completely determined by the internal anal sphincter. To actually measure basal tone the catheter inserted can be withdrawn either step-by-step or by a slow pull-through technique with a withdrawal device. The normal length of the high-pressure zone ranges from 2 to 5 cm, with a mean length of 3.5 cm [16, 23]. Because of the complex anatomy of the anal canal, the pressure varies along the length of the anal canal. In the proximal anal canal, dorsal pressures are higher than those recorded anteriorly [5, 6]. This has to be ascribed to the activity of the puborectalis muscle. In the mid-anus pressure is equally distributed over the circumference and in the lower anal canal pressure is greater anteriorly. Putting aside these influences, pressure can be divided into two patterns: the so-called slow-wave pattern with a frequency of 10 to 20 per minute and fluctuations of 5 to 25 cm H_2O, and the less frequently observed ultra-slow-wave pattern with a frequency of less than 3 per minute and fluctuations of 30 to 100 cm H_2O. Most authors consider maximal resting pressure as the reference value for basal sphincter tone.

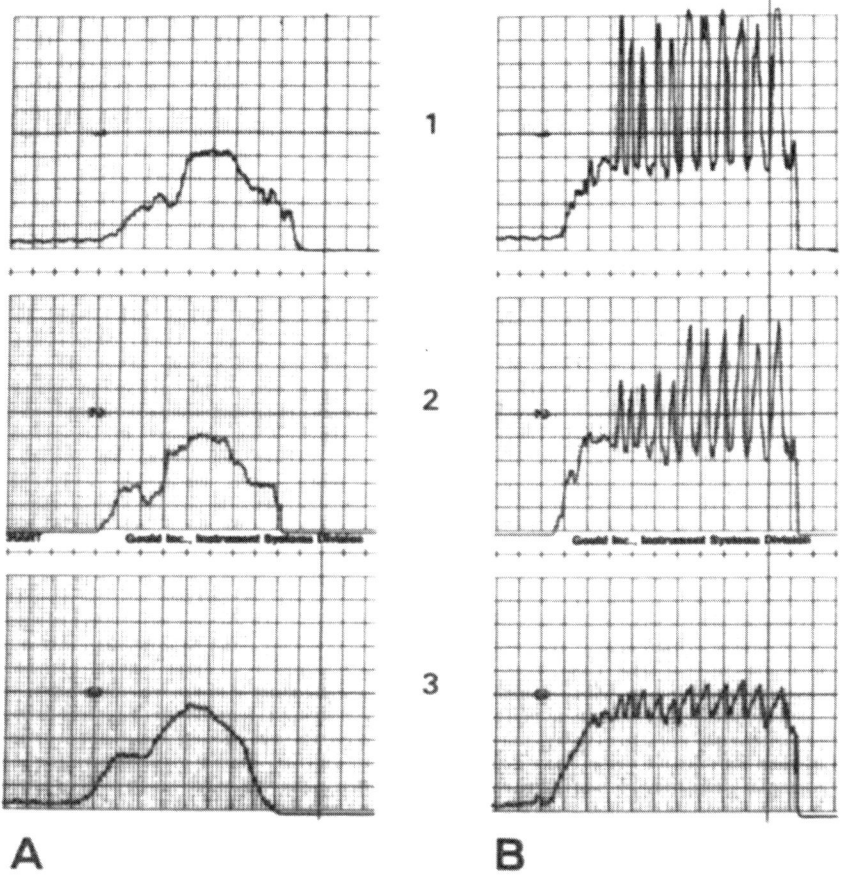

Figure 7. A. Pull through recording of anal resting pressure. B. Static recording of anal squeeze pressure. 1. Microtransducer. 2. Water-perfused catheter with low compliance pump. 3. Water-perfused catheter with high compliance pump. The water-perfused catheter with high compliance pump is not able to register quick pressure changes.

Rectal manometry

Studies of intraluminal pressures in the colon and rectum are of physiological interest and are difficult to interpret. The intra-rectal pressure in relation to intra-rectal filling or rectal compliance has been the only parameter measured which has clinical implications. The rectum has unique viscoelastic properties. Thanks to these properties the rectum has a high compliance. This enables the rectum to store large quantities of faeces without a rise in intraluminal pressure.

Technique

In most studies of intracolonic motility and intracolonic pressure a water-perfused open-tip or side-hole catheter is used. Assemblies with a closed system are prone to record artificial pressure waves [24]. A condom catheter is used for measuring rectal compliance. The rectal compliance can be tested by inflating air [25] or water in a condom catheter. The catheter has to be bench tested first and the pressure values obtained with the catheter in the rectum has to be subtracted from those obtained on bench testing.

The first percepted volume, during filling of the balloon, is called the threshold volume. This is a crude measure of rectal sensitivity. The maximal tolerated volume is another important parameter which is low in incontinent patients and high or sometimes unrecordable in megacolon.

Normal patterns of intra-rectal manometry

The intra-rectal pressure is the sum of the intra-abdominal pressure, the contractile force of the rectal wall, and the elasticity of the wall. The respiratory movements and pressure waves of about 1 kPa are easily recognised. The rectum produces the same movement and pressure pattern as the rest of the large bowel. There are two types of movement: segmenting contractions, throughout the day, and propulsive contractions, about four times a day. Intra-luminal pressure recordings cannot discriminate between the two, but 90% of the motor activity is caused by segmenting contractions [26]. During colonic contractions pressure can rise to about 8 kPa. Propulsive activity is not correlated with the intraluminal pressure pattern. Increases in intraluminal pressure are mainly due to segmenting contractions and means a slowing transit [27].

The unit most used for expressing the colonic activity is the Motor Index, i.e., the product of percentage of time in a period of pressure rise and the mean amplitude of the pressure waves [28].

Rectal compliance and volume

The pressure/volume relation or compliance has proved to be of clinical importance, since the compliance and maximal tolerated volume in the rectum are correlated to defaecation frequency and the subjective feeling of urgency [29, 30]. The maximal tolerated volume and rectal compliance are lowered in inflammatory bowel disease and in radiation injury. Normal values for rectal compliance are in the region of 5 (1.95–5.25) cc/cm H_2O [28].

Clinical application of ano-rectal manometry

Indication for anal and rectal manometry can be grouped into three different categories.

Diagnostic application

The combination of anal and rectal manometry has a place in assessing patients with faecal incontinence. It has also been performed in connection with defaecography and electromyography. It is inappropriate to decide on treatment based on manometry only, without taking defaecography and electromyography into consideration. Ano-rectal manometry is often helpful in patients with constipation, especially when there is suspicion of Hirschsprung's disease. Hirschsprung's disease must be excluded by biopsy if the recto-anal inhibitory reflex is absent. Less conclusive data are obtained with manometry in patients with the so called spastic pelvic floor syndrome and other less well defined causes of constipation. In patients with anal fissure and haemorrhoids, anal and rectal manometry play a role to selecting those patients suitable for treatment by anal dilatation or sphincterotomy. These patients should not be treated by anal dilatation if resting anal pressures are low.

Therapeutic application

Anal manometry can be used to reinforce biofeedback training in the treatment of incontinence and constipation. For a detailed description of the method and the results obtained, see Chapter 3.6.

Research application

There is an overlap between anal and rectal manometry performed for diagnostic and research purposes. Research interests are the main reasons for performing manometry before and after post-anal repair, posterior rectopexy and sphincter reconstruction. Such data are important, so that poor risk factors can be identified pre-operatively. The use of ano-rectal manometry may also be used as a means of selecting patients for ileo-rectal anastomosis after previous subtotal colectomy with end-ileostomy and for ileo-anal reservoir following restorative proctocolectomy. Anal manometry is, in fact, less useful than assessment of rectal and pouch compliance since patients with relatively low anal pressures can be fully continent, whereas apparently normal values on preoperative manometry may be associated with post-operative incontinence [7].

Summary

Anal and rectal manometry play an important role in the evaluation of patients with disordered defaecation and other ano-rectal pathology. However, without the addition of defaecography and electromyography, the evaluation of these patients is incomplete. The water-perfused catheter with a low compliance pump is the most valuable method of measuring anal pressure profiles. Any data obtained must be interpreted with reference to normal, age and control values registered with the same equipment.

References

1. Gowers WR. 1877. The automatic action of the sphincter ani. Proc Royal Soc Med 26: 77.
2. Dent J, Dodds WJ, Friedman RH et al. 1980. Mechanisms of gastroesophageal reflux in recumbent asymptomatic human subjects. J Clin Invest 65: 256–267.
3. Kerremans LD. 1969. Morphological and Physiological aspects of anal continence and defaecation. Bruxelles; Presse Académiques Européennes SC. Editions Arsica.
4. Read NW. 1985. Anorectal manometry: techniques in health and ano-rectal disease. In: Coloproctology and the pelvic floor, Henry MM, Swash M. (eds) London; Butterworths: 65–87.
5. Collins CD, Bron BH, Whittaker GE, Duthie HL. 1969. New method of measuring forces in the anal canal. Gut 10: 160–163.
6. Taylor BM, Brown BH, Whittaker GE, Duthie HL. 1984. Longitudinal and radial variations of pressure in the human anal sphincter. Gastroenterology 86: 693–697.
7. Kuypers JHC. 1982. Anal manometry, its applications and indications. The Neth J Surg 34: 153–158.
8. Hill JR, Kelly ML, Schlegel JF. 1960. Pressure profile of the rectum and anus of healthy persons. Dis Colon Rectum 3: 203–209.
9. Lydon SB, Dodds WJ, Hogan WJ, Arndorfer RC. 1975. The effect of manometric assembly diameter on intraluminal esophageal pressure recording. Dig Dis 20: 968–970.
10. Baeten CGMI. 1985. Haemorrhoids, evaluation of methods of treatment. Thesis. Maastricht.
11. Hancock BD. 1977. The internal sphincter and anal fissure. Br J Surg 64: 92–95.
12. Kramer AEJL, Teulings H. 1987. Instrumentatie voor klinisch urodynamische metingen: Aanbevelingen ICS-commissie. Medische Technologie 1.
13. Forcheri V, Dai Bò R, Caldart M, Marshall M. 1984. A quick and simple method of anal manometry. Coloproctology 6: 166–167.
14. Blessing H. 1984. The value of pull-through manometry employing a microtransducer in anal emergencies. Coloproctology 6: 152–155.
15. Blessing H. 1985. How much information does anal pull-through manometry using a microtransducer provide? Coloproctology 7: 229–233.
16. Varma JS, Smith AN. 1984. Ano-rectal profilometry with the microtransducer. Br J Surg 71: 867–869.
17. Jonas U, Klotter HJ. 1978. Study of three urethral pressure recording devices: theoretical considerations. Urological Research 6: 119–125.
18. Arndorfer RC, Stef JJ, Dodds WJ, Linehan JH, Hogan WJ. 1977. Improved infusion system for intraluminal esophageal manometry. Gastroenterology 73: 23–27.
19. Kuypers JHC. 1981. Over de perianale fistel. Thesis. Nijmegen.

20. Schweiger M. 1982. Functionelle Analsphincteruntersuchungen. Springer-Verlag Berlin Heidelberg New York 27.
21. Benneth RC, Duthie HL. 1964. The functional importance of the internal anal sphincter. Br J Surg 51: 355–357.
22. Duthie HL, Watts JM. 1965. Contribution of the external anal sphincter to the pressure zone in the anal canal. Gut 6: 64–68.
23. Nivratvong S, Stern H, Fryd DS. 1981. The length of the anal canal. Dis Colon Rectum 24: 600–601.
24. Misiewicz JJ. 1984. Human colonic motility. In: Basic Science in Gastroenterology. Polak JM, Bloom SR, Wright NA, Butler AG. Eds. Glaxo Group Research Limited. Royal Postgraduate School: 325–333.
25. Ihre T. 1974. Studies on anal function in continent and incontinent patients. Scand J Gastroenterol 9 (suppl 25): 1–64.
26. Lanfranchi GA. 1983. Motor functions and dysfunctions of the large bowel and the rectum. Coloproctology 5: 19–22.
27. Haddad H, Devroede-Bertrand G. 1981. Large bowel motility disorders. Med Clin North Am 65: 1377–1395.
28. Roe AM, Bartolo DCC, Mortensen NJMcC. 1986. Diagnosis and surgical management of intractible constipation. Br J Surg 73: 854–861.
29. Suzuki H, Matsumoto K, Amano S, Fujioka M, Honzumi M. 1980. Ano-rectal pressure and rectal compliance after low anterior resection. Br J Surg 67: 655–657.
30. Waever RM, Keighley MRB. 1986. Measurement of rectal capacity in the assessment of patients for colectomy and ileo-rectal anastomosis in Crohn's colitis. Dis Colon Rectum 29: 433–445.

1.2 Electromyography and nerve latency studies

S.J. SNOOKS & M. SWASH

Introduction

Pelvic floor disorders (Table 1) are a common cause of disability and distress often resulting in faecal incontinence especially in women, but hitherto their pathogenesis has not been well understood. We have found that these disorders are associated, in varying degree, with clinical, electrophysiological and histological features of chronic partial denervation in the muscles of the pelvic floor, especially in the puborectalis and levator ani muscles, and in the external anal and periurethral striated sphincter muscles [1–7]. These studies have led us to develop a unifying approach to understanding the pathogenesis of this

Table 1. Results of single fibre electromyography (SFEMG) studies, of pudendal nerve terminal motor latency (PNTML) and of fibre density (FD) measurements in various pelvic floor disorders.

Disorder	n	PNTML (SD)	(%)	FD (EAS)	Mean age	Mean symptom duration (yr)
Control	20	1.9 (0.2)	–	1.5 (0.16)	45	–
ARI	20	2.6 (0.8)*	80	2.1 (0.3)*	52	5
ARI + CRP	20	2.8 (0.5)*	80	1.9 (0.2)*	55	3
DI	20	2.7 (0.5)*	80	2.0 (0.3)*	60	7
SRUS	20	2.3 (0.3)*	60	1.7 (0.3)*	23	2
ASD	20	2.2 (0.4)*	60	1.7 (0.3)*	30	1
CONS	24	2.2 (0.3)*	50	1.6 (0.2)	42	2

ARI: ano-rectal incontinence.
DI: double incontinence.
CRP: complete rectal prolapse.
SRUS: solitary rectal ulcer syndrome.
ASD: anterior sphincter division due to vaginal delivery.
CONS: constipation.
EAS: external anal sphincter.
*: difference from control group ($p<0.01$; Wilcoxon test).

group of disorders that has implications for diagnosis, investigation and management, and also for prevention.

In order to illustrate this approach we present the results of our investigations in the six common types of pelvic floor disorder (Table 1). The application of electromyography and nerve latency studies are emphasized throughout.

Patients

Six groups of patients, consisting of 124 women have been studied (Table 2). These comprised 20 patients with idiopathic ano-rectal incontinence, 20 with ano-rectal incontinence associated with complete rectal prolapse, 20 with incontinence of both faeces and urine (double incontinence), 20 with solitary rectal ulcer syndrome, 20 with division of the anterior part of the external anal sphincter, associated with ano-rectal incontinence, that had occurred during difficult vaginal delivery, and 24 with severe and intractable constipation. Ano-rectal incontinence was defined as the inadvertent passage of formed faeces. Urinary incontinence consisted of genuine stress incontinence confirmed by video cystometrography. The diagnosis of solitary rectal ulcer syndrome was confirmed by biopsy. Constipation was defined as the passage of faeces less than twice per week during a period of more than two years [8, 9]. Some of these patients have been reported previously [3, 4, 6].

Twenty women without ano-rectal abnormality, who had not experienced vaginal delivery, served as controls. In addition, the results in 9 patients with cauda equina lesions [10] provided validation of our electrophysiological procedures for the assessment of abnormalities in the proximal part of the innervation of the pelvic sphincter muscles.

Table 2. Motor latencies recorded in the puborectalis (PR) and external anal sphincter (EAS) muscles after supramaximal stimulation at L1 and L4 vertebral levels in idiopathic ano-rectal incontinence (ARI) and cauda equina lesions (CEL). The ratio between the motor latencies from L1/L4 stimulation sites, termed the spinal latency ratio (SLR) is also shown.

Disorder	n	PR		EAS		SLR
		L1 (ms)	L4 (ms)	L1 (ms)	L4 (ms)	L1/L4
Control	20	4.8 (0.4)	3.7 (0.5)	5.5 (0.4)	4.4 (0.4)	1.3 (0.1)
ARI	7	6.2 (1.4)*	3.5 (0.9)	6.0 (0.9)*	4.5 (0.7)*	1.8 (0.2)*
CEL	9	6.5 (1.1)*	3.8 (0.9)	7.2 (0.8)*	4.6 (0.9)*	1.7 (0.3)*

* Difference from control group ($p < 0.01$: Wilcoxon test).

Electromyography

Conventional concentric EMG

The electrical activity generated by the external sphincter was first studied by Beck [11] who recorded potentials by means of steel electrodes. Floyd and Walls [12] investigated the external sphincter in man using surface electrodes which comprised 1 cm diameter silver/silver chloride discs which were applied to the peri-anal skin.

Surface electrodes cause minimal interference to the muscle and are consequently readily tolerated by patients. However, the potentials recorded are summated from multiple motor units. The electrical activity generated by the active contraction of nearby adductor and gluteal muscle groups may be indistinguishable from potentials arising from the external sphincter complex.

For these reasons we prefer to use bipolar concentric needle electrodes since the summated potentials from only a limited (up to approximately 30) number of muscle fibres lying within the vicinity of the electrode tip are recorded [13]. The electrodes (Medelec EL75M) consist of an outer cannula 3 cm long, one end of which is pointed and bevelled to facilitate entry through the skin and an inner core of wire separated from the cannula by an insulating layer (Figure 1). The potential difference between the bare tip of the centre wire and the outer cannula over an area of $0.22 \, mm^2$ is recorded using this technique. Since the amplitude of the recorder potentials within the external sphincter and pelvic floor muscles is of the order of 50 mV to 2 mV it is necessary to amplify the signals before display on an oscilloscope or before a permanent recording is made.

With the patient lying in the left lateral position a ground electrode is strapped to the uppermost thigh and recordings made in the resting state, during voluntary contraction and during defaecation. The needle is inserted into the external sphincter without local anaesthetic; in addition, recordings are sometimes made from the puborectalis muscle. In the latter case the needle is guided into position from the perineal skin by digital palpation of the muscle in the upper posterior part of the anal canal.

In the normal resting state continuous or 'basal' action potentials will be obtained in both muscles [12]. This phenomenon is not usually displayed by skeletal muscle which is characteristically electrically silent at rest. It probably arises as a result of a spinal reflex [14]. During voluntary contraction there is a burst of activity which is the consequence of increased frequency of motor unit firing and recruitment of new motor units [15]. In contrast, during defaecation, reflex inhibition of electrical activity occurs followed by brief periods of greatly increased activity at the completion of this act.

The earliest neurological assessment of the pelvic floor in certain physiologi-

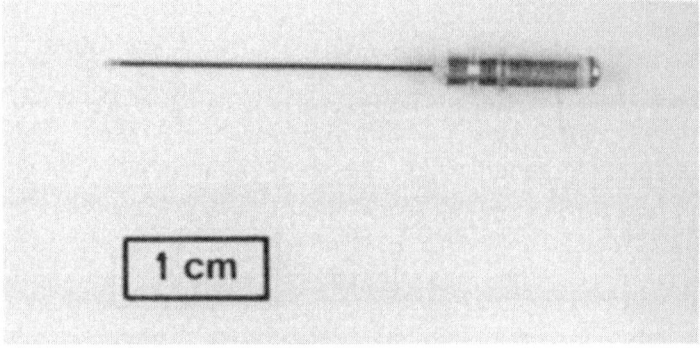

Figure 1. A concentric EMG electrode.

cal abnormalities of this region was made using conventional electromyography [16]. In patients with idiopathic incontinence the usual finding is a marked reduction in interference pattern and resting electrical activity. This is generalized for any part of the external sphincter or pelvic floor sampled. Again, this is not an easy technique to quantify although this is possible [17]. Conventional EMG is of greater importance in sphincter mapping in patients who have suffered traumatic division of the external sphincter complex. Electromyographic exploration of the perineum may assist identification of the retracted divided ends of the sphincter. This information may be of considerable assistance to the surgeon when sphincter repair is being contemplated. It is also useful in the pre- and post-operative assessment of congenital abnormalities of the anus.

Single fibre EMG

The individual motor unit potentials recorded with a concentric needle electrode are generated by the muscle fibres of individual motor units [18]. The amplitude and shape of the motor unit potential is determined by the number of muscle fibres within the recording area of the concentric needle electrode. This method thus has limitations because little information is gained with respect to the individual elements generating the motor unit potential. As a result of these inadequacies the concept of single fibre EMG has been developed [18].

This technique identifies the muscle action potential from a single muscle fibre, by employing an electrode of 25 to 30 μm in diameter. The technique provides a means of assessing innervation and reinnervation of skeletal muscle under investigation. The assessment can be made quantitatively by means of the fibre density which represents the mean of the number of muscle fibres from one motor unit within the uptake area of the electrode in 20 different

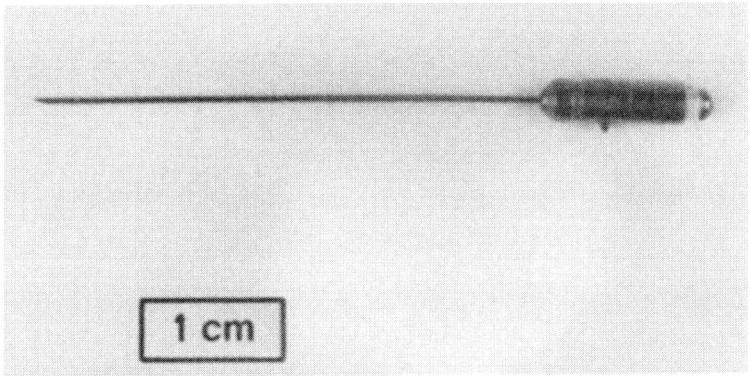

Figure 2. A single fibre EMG electrode.

electrode positions. If the fibre density is raised then this may be used as an index of collateral sprouting and reinnervation of muscle fibres within the muscle under study [19].

Collateral axonal sprouting and reinnervation of denervated muscles takes place from neighbouring healthy axons [20]. The external sphincter behaves similarly to other skeletal muscles in that its fibre density rises slightly after the age of 60 years, indicating that the innervation becomes damaged [2].

The technique as we have applied it to the external sphincter involves the insertion of a Miller-Abbott balloon into the rectum, inflating it with 30 ml of air and applying 150 g of traction. Using this technique the rate of motor unit firing is increased, thereby facilitating the identification of motor unit activity. This should be assessed in at least 20 differing sites in the external sphincter complex. In our laboratory a motor unit potential is only analysed if its rise time is faster than 300 ms and its amplitude is greater than 100 μV. The technique employs standard EMG equipment and single fibre EMG electrodes (Figure 2), using a low frequency band pass filter of 500 Hz in the amplifier [18]. It requires a moderate degree of practice before satisfactory results can be obtained.

This was one of the first truly objective quantitative means of assessing skeletal muscle function and in our laboratory has become one of the most important investigations in the assessment of denervation of the pelvic floor musculature. In the majority of patients with idiopathic incontinence the fibre density is raised, consistent with reinnervation. Pelvic floor denervation is not a feature confined to primary (idiopathic) faecal incontinence, but may occur secondary to certain generalised neurological disorders or to localised damage to the cauda equina. Traumatic injury to the pelvic floor may also be associated with a degree of denervation of the external sphincter and puborectalis muscles. A raised single fibre EMG fibre density in these muscles would

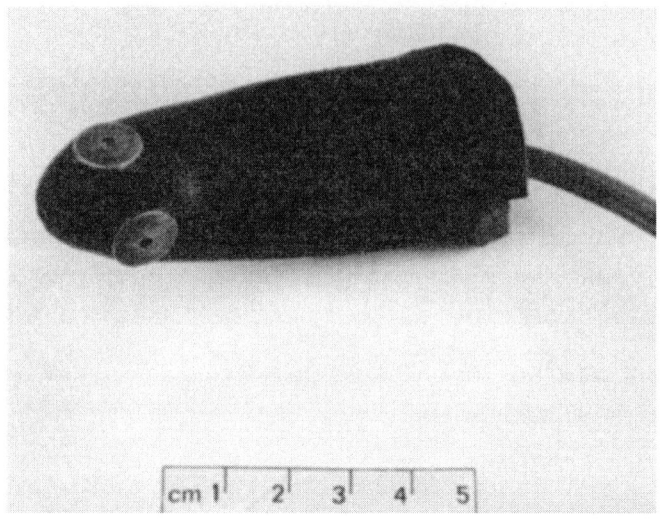

Figure 3. Transrectal glove for recording the contraction response of the puborectalis after L1 and L4 spinal stimulation.

suggest a poor functional result following a simple surgical repair of the sphincters.

Nerve stimulation techniques

Spinal stimulation

Transcutaneous electrical stimulation of the spinal cord was first achieved by Merton et al. [21]. The patient lies in the left lateral position and a stimulus of 700 to 1000 volts (duration 0.5 ms) is applied to the spine initially at the level of L1 and repeated at level L4. The stimulus electrode comprises two 1 cm diameter gauze pads 5 cm apart. The pads are soaked in physiological saline and applied vertically across the spine; the cathode is placed caudally. The induced response within the pelvic floor can be detected either by a surface anal fingerglove electrode (Figure 3) or by an intramuscular needle electrode. We have found that it can be important to differentiate between the puborectalis and external sphincter since it appears these muscles have separate innervations [22]. In the normal individual the differing motor latencies to the two muscles following spinal stimulation support this contention.

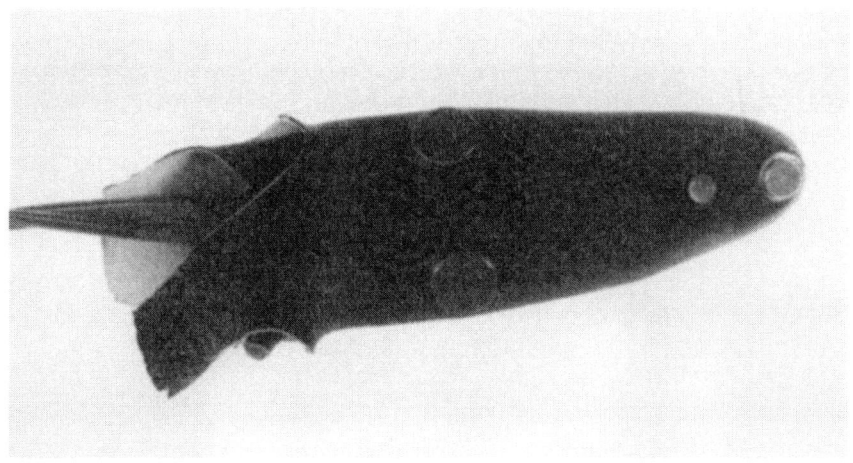

Figure 4. The pudendal nerve stimulator.

Pudendal nerve terminal motor latency: transrectal stimulation technique

This method which we have employed for determining the pudendal nerve terminal motor latency was developed from the technique of electro-ejaculation for use in patients with impotence [23]. The device consists of two stimulating electrodes situated at the tip of a rubber finger stall; two recording surface electrodes are incorporated into its base (Figure 4). The anode is 5 mm and the cathode is less than 1 mm in diameter to improve the accuracy of stimulus localisation. The recording electrodes consist of two 1 cm diameter metal plates separated by 1 cm located side by side 3 cm from the cathode so that they are at the base of the examiner's finger when the device is in use.

The patient lies in the left lateral position with a ground electrode strapped to the uppermost thigh. A rectal examination is performed with a rubber finger stall and the tip (stimulating electrode) is brought into contact with the ischial spine of either side. A square wave stimulus of 0.1 ms duration and 30 volt amplitude is delivered. The oscilloscope tracing is examined for evidence of contraction, as detected in the external anal sphincter by the surface electrode, indicating accurate localisation of the pudendal nerve. As soon as this has been achieved a supra-maximal stimulus (usually of the order of 50 volts) is delivered and the latency measured on each side.

These have been developed from the initial histological studies which demonstrated that in many patients with idiopathic incontinence the pelvic floor musculature showed features consistent with denervation [1]. Many of these patients show an increased pudendal nerve terminal motor latency [24] so indicating localised damage to this portion of the nerve. Such neurological

24

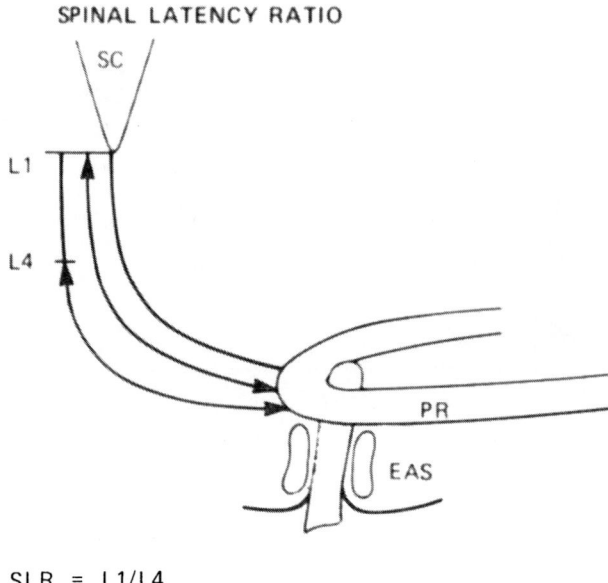

SPINAL LATENCY RATIO

SC

L1

L4

PR

EAS

SLR = L1/L4

Figure 5. Concept of recording spinal latencies at L1 and L4 with the transrectal glove in position for recording the puborectalis muscles' contraction response. The spinal latency ratio (L1/L4: SLR) can thus be determined.

damage has usually (80% of patients) been inflicted by traumatic childbirth often associated with stretch-induced injury due to abnormal degrees of descent of the pelvic floor [25]. In some nulliparous women the syndrome seems to be associated with long-continued straining at stool, perineal descent and intractable constipation [1, 24, 25].

Recently, it has become possible to investigate the central (cauda equina) component of the motor innervation of the pelvic floor by the technique of transcutaneous spinal stimulation. The latency of the motor unit action potential to the external sphincter (or puborectalis) following stimulation of the spinal cord at L1 and L4 is compared to the pudendal nerve terminal latency. Our results indicate that incontinence in some patients results from a central cause (e.g. spinal stenosis) [10]. In these patients the difference in latencies from L1 and L4 is considerably increased compared with control groups. In some patients the pudendal nerve terminal latency may also be increased suggesting that a mixed lesion may be responsible.

Summary of methods

Single fibre EMG is used to determine the fibre density, a measure of the packing density of muscle fibres in individual motor units that can be used as

SPINAL LATENCY

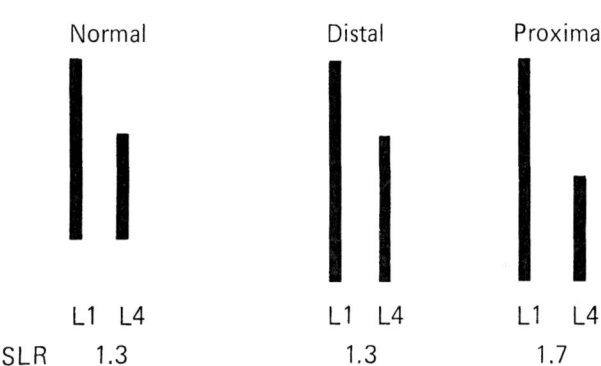

Figure 6. Normal, distal and proximal L1 and L4 spinal latencies demonstrating an inverse in the SLR when cauda equina conduction is slowed and no change in the SLR when the lesion is distal and both L1 and L4 latencies are similarly increased.

an index of reinnervation, in the external anal sphincter and puborectalis muscles [2]. The pudendal nerve terminal motor latency (PNTML) is used to assess motor conduction in the distal part of the pudendal innervation of the external anal sphincter muscle [3, 4, 24, 26]. Transcutaneous stimulation of sacral spinal motor nerve roots in the cauda equina is used to assess motor conduction within the spinal canal, and in the proximal parts of the innervations of the external anal sphincter and puborectalis muscles [10, 25]. Motor latencies are measured from supramaximal stimulation at the L1 and L4 vertebral levels. The difference between these two measured motor latencies is increased when there is a lesion in the motor roots in the cauda equina [10], and the ratio of the two latencies can be used as a simple index of the presence of a proximal or distal lesion in the innervation of the external anal sphincter, puborectalis, or periurethral striated sphincter musculature, depending on the recording site chosen [3, 4, 7, 10, 24] (Figure 5, 6).

Since the puborectalis is particularly relevant to faecal continence [1, 5, 27, 28] assessment of the innervation of this muscle is especially important. However, the innervation of this muscle probably differs from that of the external anal sphincter muscle [2] being derived, not from the pudendal nerves, but from direct pelvic branches of the motor roots of S3 and S4 [22]. Since it is not possible to stimulate these nerves within the pelvis, the innervation of this muscle can only be assessed by latency measurements from transcutaneous stimulation of the sacral nerve roots in the cauda equina [10, 26].

The Wilcoxon Rank Sum test was used for comparison of data in the various patient groups.

Results

In each of the seven groups of patients with pelvic floor disorders the mean PNTML was increased compared with the control group ($p<0.01$), but the PNTML was normal in the patients with cauda equina lesions (Table 1). In the latter group of patients motor nerve conduction was slowed in the proximal part of the innervation of these muscles, as assessed by the motor latencies from spinal stimulation at the L1 and L4 vertebral levels. Slowing of motor conduction in the proximal innervation of the pelvic sphincter muscles, in addition to the distal abnormality shown by the PNTML measurements (Table 2), is also found in 12% of patients with idiopathic ano-rectal incontinence [4].

The PNTML was more abnormal in the patients with ano-rectal incontinence than in the other patients. For example, in the patients with intractable constipation the mean PNTML was 2.2 ms, but in the patients with ano-rectal incontinence it was greater than 2.5 ms, i.e., 80% greater than normal. Similarly, the mean fibre density in the external anal sphincter muscle was significantly greater in the patients with incontinence, in whom it was 1.9 or more, than in the patients in whom continence was not compromised, in whom it was normal or nearly normal (Table 1).

Discussion

The clinical features of these different types of pelvic floor disorder overlap, particularly in the presence of weakness of the pelvic musculature, including the sphincter muscles, and the presence of perineal descent or straining. These features are accompanied by histological [1, 5] and electrophysiological [2–4, 6–8, 10, 25, 28] evidence of chronic partial denervation of these muscles and of damage to their nerve supply [26]. These abnormalities are most evident in patients with incontinence. Indeed, incontinence is not found when the single fibre EMG fibre density is less than 1.9, and the PNTML is less than 2.5 (Table 1), except in patients in whom the cause of pelvic sphincter denervation is situated in the cauda equina or in the nerves in the pelvis, in whom the PNTML may be normal and spinal stimulation is required to demonstrate the nerve lesion (Table 2).

The overlapping features of these disorders suggest that they are causally related. Damage to the innervation of the pelvic floor muscles can arise from a combination of factors acting directly or indirectly (Figure 7).

Direct factors

Occult pudendal nerve damage, although usually symptomless, is common

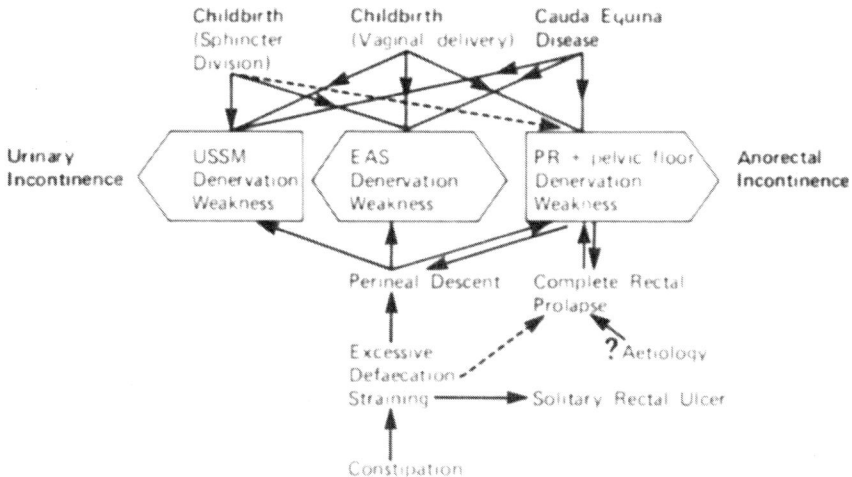

Figure 7. Pathogenesis of pelvic floor disorders. (USSM = urethral striated sphincter musculature; PR = puborectalis)

after uncomplicated vaginal delivery [29]. In some women, particularly in multiparous women, this pudendal nerve damage persists, although in most primiparous women it rapidly recovers [29]. Multiple vaginal deliveries, or difficult vaginal delivery, are common features in the past histories of women presenting with incontinence [25, 27, 28, 30], and this has led us to suggest that occult injury during childbirth is the major direct factor leading to damage to the innervation of the pelvic sphincters [1, 5, 26, 28], and so to weakness of these muscles.

However, incontinence usually develops many years after childbirth, rather than immediately, indicating that there are other contributory factors. One of these, present in about 12% of patients with idiopathic ano-rectal incontinence, is damage to the motor nerve roots of S3 and S4 in the cauda equina [4] often due to coincidental disc disease, or stenosis of the spinal canal from osteoarthritis. This may be the sole cause of denervation of the pelvic sphincter musculature [10], but it is more commonly a contributory cause in patients in whom there is also damage to the distal parts of the innervation of these muscles, initiated in childbirth [22, 24–29].

Indirect factors

Constipation and a history of repeated defaecation straining are frequently noted in patients presenting with idiopathic ano-rectal incontinence [1, 5, 27]. These functional abnormalities are of uncertain and perhaps multiple causes but they are often associated with perineal descent on straining [25, 29]. The latter may itself cause damage to the innervation of the pelvic floor sphincter musculature because of the repeated stretch injury to these nerves that may occur during this downward movement of the pelvic floor [6, 26, 31]. Patients with excessive perineal descent have an obtuse ano-rectal angle, with loss of the post-defaecation closure reflex, and are thus predisposed to rectal prolapse [3, 27, 31]. Rectal prolapse is also often associated with faecal incontinence, but patients with this combination of problems show similar electrophysiolog-ical abnormalities to those found in patients with ano-rectal incontinence alone [3, 31] (Table 1). The inter-relation of these features and of solitary rectal ulcer syndrome to incontinence is shown in Figure 7. These indirect factors thus lead to further damage to the innervation of the pelvic sphincters and pelvic floor muscles. However, constipation, defaecation straining and pelvic floor descent may themselves follow pelvic floor damage initiated during childbirth, thus starting a cycle of events culminating in severe functional disturbance.

Pelvic floor disorders commonly present after the menopause [26, 28], a feature suggesting that hormonal factors may be important. This concept is supported by a structural sexual dimorphism found in the human levator ani muscle. In this muscle, in women, the Type 1 muscle fibres are larger than the Type 2 fibres, although in all other skeletal muscles, as in men, Type 1 fibres are slightly smaller than Type 2 fibres [32]. The functional significance of this feature in this muscle is unknown, but Type 1 muscle fibres are functionally adapted for tonic activity. Age-related changes in fibre type characteristics in the pelvic floor muscles have not yet been studied.

Incontinence and the extent of electrophysiological abnormality

Ano-rectal incontinence is not likely to develop unless the fibre density in single fibre EMG studies of the external anal sphincter or the puborectalis muscles is greater than 2.5, or the PNTML is greater than 1.8 (Table 1). These abnormalities imply a considerable degree of damage to the innervation of these muscles. Our earlier histological studies showed that these muscles were very severely damaged in patients biopsied during attempted surgical correc-tion of incontinence [1, 5], indicating that the functional reserve in these muscles had been exceeded.

Finally, it must be recognised that damage to the innervation of the pelvic floor sphincter muscles is not the only cause of sphincter weakness leading to incontinence [30], although it is by far the commonest. Our histological studies suggested that about 80% of patients with ano-rectal incontinence had dener-vation of these muscles, but the histological features of some of the muscles examined [1, 5] showed end-stage disease so that the underlying pattern characteristic of denervation and reinnervation could not be recognised. Our electrophysiological investigations not only indicate that neurogenic sphincter damage is the usual cause of this syndrome of stress ano-rectal incontinence, and probably also of stress urinary incontinence, but suggest that there is a relationship between the functional pelvic floor disorders (Table 1), and faecal incontinence [26].

References

1. Parks AG, Swash M, Urich H. 1977. Sphincter denervation in ano-rectal incontinence and rectal prolapse. Gut 18: 656–665.
2. Neill ME, Swash M. 1980. Increased motor unit fibre density in the external anal sphincter muscle in ano-rectal incontinence; a single fibre EMG study. J Neurol Neurosurg Psych 43: 343–347.
3. Snooks SJ, Henry MM, Swash M. 1985. Ano-rectal incontinence and rectal prolapse; differential assessment of the puborectalis and external anal sphincter muscles. Gut 26: 470–477.
4. Snooks SJ, Henry MM, Swash M. 1985. Abnormalities in central and peripheral nerve conduction in ano-rectal incontinence. J Roy Soc Med 78: 294–300.
5. Beersiek F, Parks AG, Swash M. 1979. Pathogenesis of pelvic floor disorders; a histometric study of the anal sphincter musculature. J Neurol Sci 42: 111–127.
6. Snooks SJ, Barnes PRH, Swash M. 1984. Damage to the innervation of the voluntary anal and periurethral sphincter musculature in incontinence; an electrophysiological study. J Neurol Neurosurg Psychiatry 47: 1269–1273.
7. Snooks SJ, Swash M. 1984. Abnormalities of the urethral striated sphincter musculature in incontinence. Br J Urol 56: 401–405.
8. Snooks SJ, Barnes PRH, Swash M, Henry MM. 1985. Damage to the innervation of the pelvic floor musculature in chronic constipation. Gastroenterology 89: 977–981.
9. Preston DM, Lennard-Jones JE. 1985. Anismus in chronic constipation. Dig Dis Sci 30: 413–418.
10. Snooks SJ, Swash M. 1986. Slowed motor conduction in the lumbosacral nerve roots in cauda equina lesions. J Neurol Neuro Surg Psych 49: 808–816.
11. Beck A. 1930. Electromyographische Untersuchungen am sphincter ani. Pfugers Arch Ges Physiol 224: 278.
12. Floyd WD, Walls EW. 1953. Electromyography of the sphincter ani externus in man. Journal of Physiology, London 122: 599–609.
13. Buchtal F. 1960. The general concept of the motor unit. Res Publ Ass Nerv Ment Dis 38: 3.
14. Parks AG, Porter NH, Hardcastle J. 1966. The syndrome of the descending perineum. Proc Roy Soc Med 59: 477–482.
15. Kerremans R. 1969. Morphological and physiological aspects of anal continence and defaecation. Editions Arscia, Brussels.
16. Porter NH. 1962. A physiological study of the pelvic floor in rectal prolapse. Ann Roy Coll Surg Engl 31: 379–401.
17. Bartolo DCC, Jarratt JA, Read MG, Donnelly TC, Read NW. 1983. The role of partial denervation of the puborectalis in idiopathic faecal incontinence. Br J Surg 70: 664–667.
18. Stalberg E, Trontelj JV. 1979. Single fibre electromyography. Old Woking, Surrey, UK. The Mirralle Press Ltd: 64.
19. Swash M, Schwartz MS. 1984. Implications of longitudinal fibre splitting in neurogenic and myopathic disorders. Springer-Verlag, London: 350.

20. Stalberg E, Thiele B. 1975. Motor unit fibre density in the extensor digitorum communis muscle. J Neurol Neurosurg Psych 38: 874–880.
21. Merton PA, Hill DK, Morton HB, Marsden CD. 1982. Scope of a technique for electrical stimulation of human brain, spinal cord and muscle. Lancet i: 597–600.
22. Percy JP, Neill ME, Swash M, Parks AG. 1981. Electrophysiological study of motor nerve supply of pelvic floor. Lancet i: 16–17.
23. Brindley GS. 1981. Electroejaculation: its technique, neurological implications and use. Neurol Neurosurg Psych 44: 9–18.
24. Kiff ES, Swash M. 1984. Slowed conduction in the pudendal nerves in idiopathic (neurogenic) faecal incontinence. Br J Surg 71: 614–616.
25. Henry MM, Parks AG, Swash M. 1982. The pelvic floor musculature in the descending perineum syndrome. Br J Surg 69: 470–472.
26. Henry MM, Swash M. 1985. Coloproctology and the Pelvic Floor. Butterworths. London.
27. Snooks SJ, Badenoch D, Tiptaft R, Swash M. 1985. Perineal nerve damage in genuine stress urinary incontinence; an electrophysiological study. Br J Urol 57: 422–426.
28. Parks AG. 1975. Ano-rectal incontinence. Proc Roy Soc Med 68: 681–690.
29. Snooks SJ, Swash M, Setchell M, Henry MM. 1984. Injury to innervation of pelvic floor sphincter musculature in childbirth. Lancet ii: 546–550.
30. Snooks SJ, Henry MM, Swash M. 1985. Obstetric sphincter division and pudendal nerve damage; a double lesion. Br J Obstet Gynaecol. In press.
31. Neill ME, Parks AG, Swash M. 1981. Physiological studies of the anal sphincter musculature in faecal incontinence and rectal prolapse. Br J Surg 68: 531–536.
32. Polgar J, Johnson M, Weightman D, Appleton D. 1973. Data on fibre size in thirty-six human muscles; an autopsy study. J Neurol Sci 19: 307–318.

1.3 Defaecography

N.R. WOMACK & N.S. WILLIAMS

Introduction

Radiology has been used to study normal and disordered ano-rectal function. The techniques employed have undergone modification and refinement in an attempt to record, as near as possible, the natural state. Such techniques can give precise anatomical information about the ano-rectum and recently the addition of simultaneous measurement of sphincteric EMG activity and intra-rectal pressure has allowed insight into the activity of the pelvic floor during voiding. However, the fact that the subject is aware that what is essentially a personal and private function is being studied and recorded means that all techniques are a compromise and record only an approximation of the natural state. This must always be remembered when interpreting the activity of muscles that are under voluntary control.

Historical background

Early investigations of rectal voiding were reported in the mid-1960s using the technique of cineradiography. From the outset the choice of contrast medium has varied. Those workers who investigated specific ano-rectal abnormalities, such as prolapse [1, 2], found that liquid barium suspensions were adequate, and convenient. Investigation of the normal physiology of continence and defaecation, however, required a semi-solid medium similar to faeces. Phillips and Edwards [3] achieved this aim by opacifying the normal colonic contents with orally ingested barium sulphate. The disadvantage of such a technique was the timing of the subsequent radiological investigation, which made this method impractical for routine clinical use. The alternative was to produce a synthetic 'stool' which could be introduced into the rectum prior to the investigation. Such a technique was first reported by Kerremans [4] who used a mixture of plasticine, talc and barium sulphate. Later workers have used similar substitutes based on potato starch [5] or rolled oats [6] to achieve a contrast medium with a semi-solid consistency.

In an attempt to simplify the procedure and make it more aesthetically acceptable to patients and staff, Preston and his colleagues [7] developed the balloon proctogram. This employed a specially shaped balloon that contained 150 ml of barium suspension. It allowed measurement of certain parameters, such as ano-rectal angle, under conditions of stress to the pelvic floor, but was found to be inferior to free contrast medium in the rectum for the study of voiding abnormalities [8].

Recently, in response to suggestions that abnormal function of the pelvic floor muscles may contribute to voiding disorders, we have developed a method to visualise the ano-rectum during voiding of a semi-solid contrast medium, whilst simultaneously measuring the EMG activity of the puborectalis and superficial parts of the external anal sphincter, and the intra-rectal pressure by radiotelemetry.

Method of defaecography

The procedure is performed without bowel preparation on the day of study. In some constipated patients enemas have been necessary on preceding days to empty the bowel.

Intra-rectal pressure is measured using a pressure-sensitive radiotelemetry capsule (RTC). This is pre-calibrated against a water manometer at 37° C. It is inserted into the rectum before the contrast medium, the signal from the capsule is received by an omnidirectional aerial strapped over the subject's sacrum.

Electromyographic activity from the puborectalis and superficial components of the external anal sphincter is recorded by the insertion of fine stainless steel wire electrodes.

The contrast medium is prepared by heating 70 g of rolled oats with 150 g of barium sulphate and 300 ml of water. 250–300 ml of this paste is then introduced into the rectum, via a proctoscope, using a wide tipped syringe. The subject is then seated on a radiolucent commode to void the contrast (Figure 1).

Synchronisation and storage of data

Integrated EMG and pressure data are digitised by a microcomputer. The computer is programmed to store the data on floppy disc and to produce a graphic display of the data. The computer graphics are synchronized with the radiological image, the composite picture then being stored on videotape. A

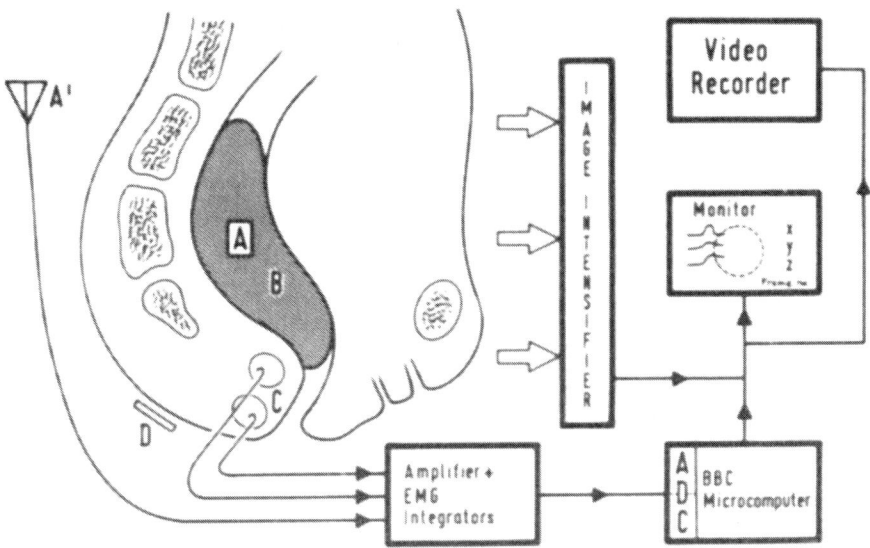

Figure 1. Diagrammatic representation of the methods used for defaecography. (Key A = Pressure sensitive radiotelemetry capsule; A¹ = Omnidirectional antenna; B = Semi-solid contrast medium; D = 3 cm radio-opaque marker on skin; ADC = Analogue to digital converter).

hard copy of the pressure and EMG data can be obtained from the computer at a later date (Figure 2); this greatly facilitates analysis of these data.

This method allows investigation of the following parameters:

1) ano-rectal angle at rest, straining and during voiding,
2) perineal descent during straining and voiding,
3) detection of anatomical abnormalities of the ano-rectum during voiding,
4) measurement of external anal sphincter EMG activity at rest, during maximal contraction and during voiding,
5) measurement of the rise in intra-rectal pressure associated with voiding or attempts to void.

The technique has been used to study normal individuals and patients with suspected disorders of ano-rectal function.

Mechanisms of continence and defaecation

Defaecography has revealed the functional anatomy of the ano-rectum. At rest the anal canal is flattened from side to side forming a slit in the sagittal plane [3]. There is angulation of $92° \pm 1.5$ (mean $\pm$ SEM) at the ano-rectal junction [5]. This angulation is held to be important for the maintenance of continence. It results from the activity of the puborectalis muscular sling, the

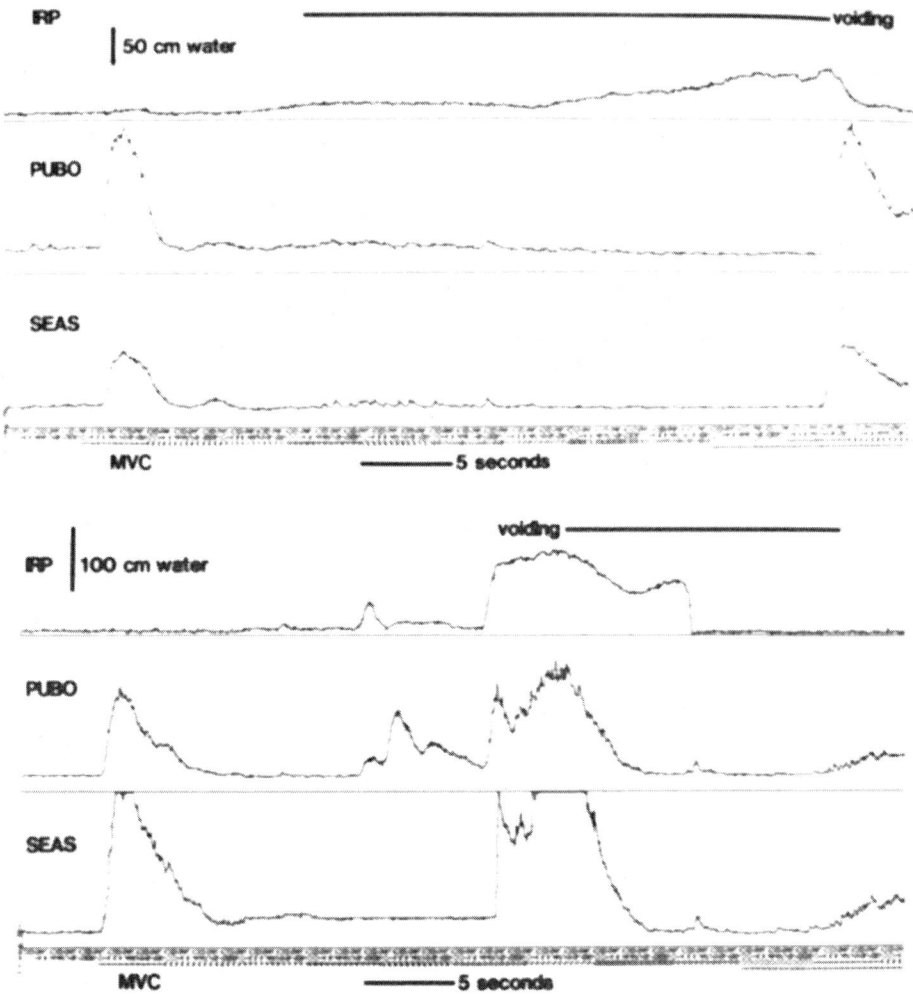

Figure 2. Printouts of intra-rectal pressure and sphincter EMG activity during voiding. A. Normal subject, voiding commences with low intra-rectal pressure and immediate inhibition of the sphincters. B. Normal subject, voiding follows a period of straining during which sphincter EMG activity is recruited. (Key IRP = Intra-rectal pressure; PUBO = Puborectalis EMG activity; SEAS = Superficial external anal sphincter EMG activity; MVC = Maximum voluntary contraction of the anal sphincters).

activity of which increases reflexly when intra-abdominal pressure rises and continence is threatened [9]. This reflex has been shown to be deficient in patients with faecal incontinence [10]. The widely accepted 'flap- valve' theory of continence [11] is not supported by the findings on defaecography, since the rectal contents are not prevented from overlying the canal by the anterior rectal mucosa.

During defaecation the pelvic floor descends and the ano-rectal angle becomes more obtuse ($137° \pm 1.5$) [5]. Pelvic floor descent should not exceed 2 cm [5]. Electromyography has shown that the activity in the sphincteric muscles, during voiding, is variable (Figure 2). Generally activity in the puborectalis is inhibited though not totally abolished. Inhibition of activity also occurs in the superficial part of the sphincter, usually to a greater degree than in the puborectalis. In a small percentage of normal subjects, however, inhibition of sphincter activity does not occur and there is either no change, or an increase in, sphincteric activity during voiding. At the end of defaecation a burst of activity in the sphincters empties the canal anal and returns the pelvic floor to the rest position. The rise in intra-rectal pressure necessary to void the contrast medium in our normal subjects was 60 cm water (50–140) median and range. The contribution of rectal contraction to the evacuation of rectal contents remains unclear at present.

Disorders of ano-rectal function

Rectal prolapse

Defaecography has been useful in the study of rectal prolapse. Some degree of perineal descent, with widening of the ano-rectal angle, is usually present at rest. Most prolapses start with an invagination of the rectal wall 6–8 cm from the ano-rectal junction. This defect is usually anteriorly placed (60%) or annular (32%) [12]. The infolding proceeds forming an intussusception (Figure 3). This may remain internal or pass through the anal canal. The final stage in the formation of a full thickness prolapse is eversion of the mucosa of the anal canal. When the prolapse is down ano-rectal angulation is lost and the ano-rectum becomes vertically disposed. The rectal prolapse frequently only develops towards the end of rectal evacuation and the investigation must therefore be continued until the rectum is empty if such a lesion is to be excluded.

The use of defaecography has necessitated a re-definition of terms regarding rectal prolapse, since demonstration of clinically occult lesions has made the accepted definition of rectal prolapse – the protrusion of part or all layers of the rectal wall through the anal orifice – inadequate. Radiologically lesions can be divided into anterior rectal wall prolapse, which may be intra-anal or extra-anal, and intussusception which may be intra-anal or extra-anal. The general term 'rectal prolapse' embraces this spectrum of conditions.

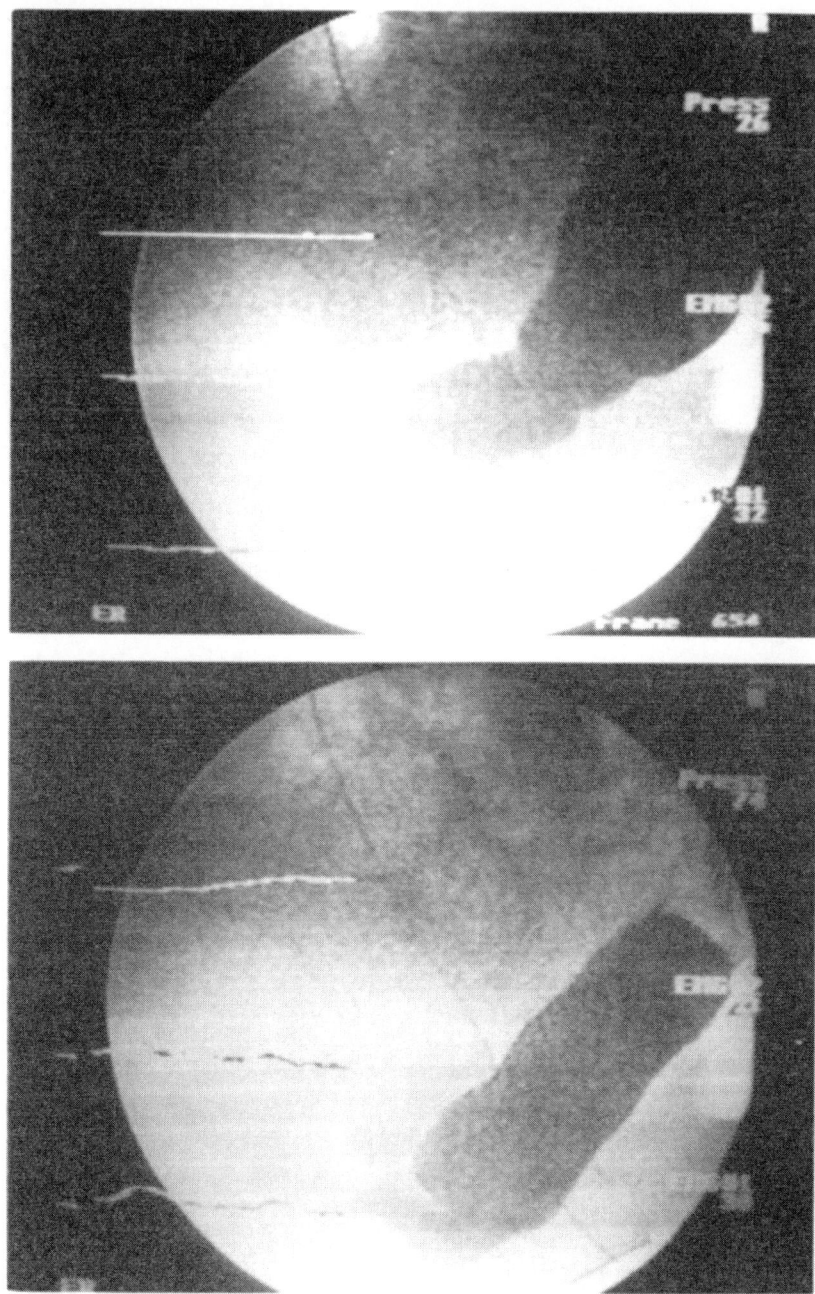

Figure 3. The development of a full thickness rectal prolapse. (Key: Upper trace – intra-rectal pressure; middle trace – puborectalis activity; lower trace – superficial external anal sphincter activity). A. The outline of the ano-rectum at rest. B. With straining, invagination of the anterior

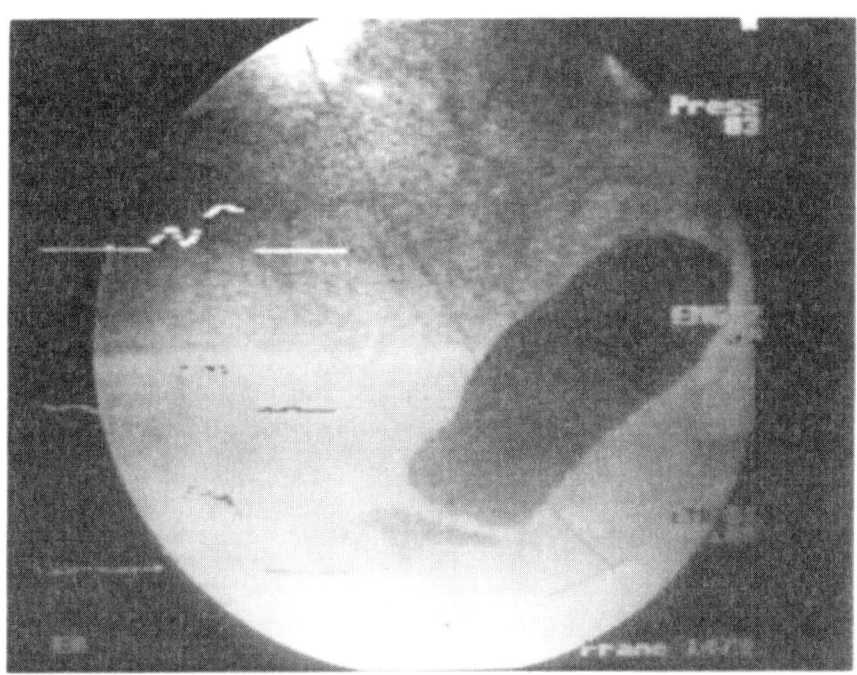

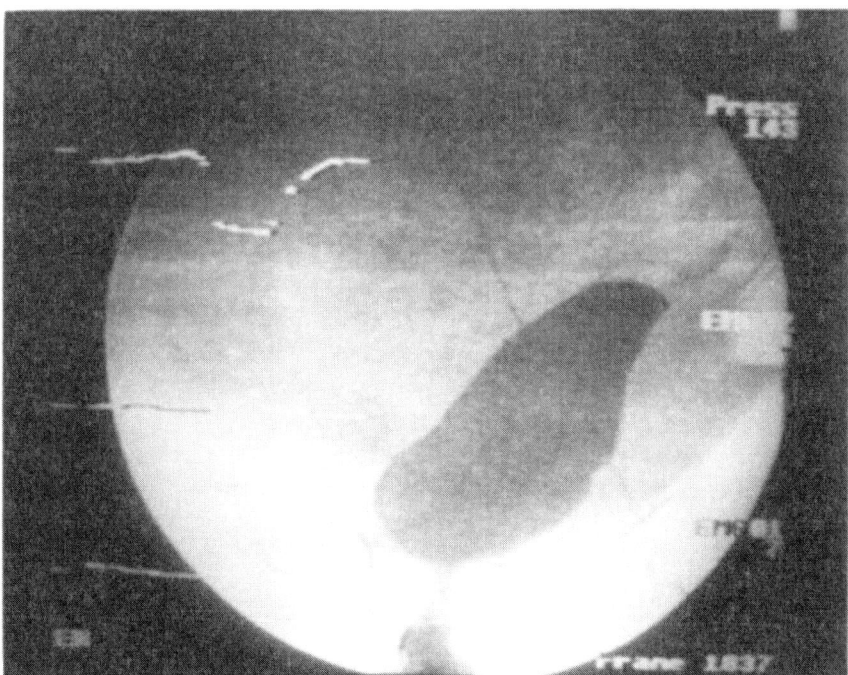

rectal wall occurs. C. with further straining, there is invagination of the anterior and posterior rectal walls. D. The invagination has passed through the anal canal and eversion of the anal mucosa has resulted in a full thickness rectal prolapse.

Solitary rectal ulcer syndrome (SRUS)

A clinical association between SRUS and rectal prolapse was noted by Madigan and Morson [13], and was emphasised by Rutter [14]. Use of defaecography has confirmed this relationship and has demonstrated a high incidence of clinically occult rectal intussusception in the these patients. In Mahieu's [15] series of 22 patients rectal prolapse was present in 17 of the 21 (81%) who voided, and in our series of 18 patients a rectal prolapse was present in 15 of the 16 (94%) patients able to void contrast. Abnormal hyperactivity of the pelvic floor muscles during straining has been described in this condition [16]. Use of our technique has confirmed the presence of such an abnormality in those patients with SRUS who describe symptoms of obstructed defaecation [17].

Du Boulay and colleagues [18] have shown that the histological changes found in the rectal mucosa in SRUS are probably caused by mucosal prolapse. However, not all patients with these histological changes develop rectal ulceration. To investigate why this should be, we have compared a group of patients with the histological changes of SRUS and rectal ulceration with a group with the histological changes alone. A high incidence of rectal prolapse (⩾89%) was present in both groups. There were three differences between the groups. The patients with rectal ulceration were younger. They demonstrated a greater degree of overactivity in their sphincters during voiding, and voiding required a greater increase in intra-rectal pressure than in the patients without ulceration (unpublished observations). This finding suggests that solitary rectal ulceration occurs when high voiding pressure and rectal prolapse combine. This situation exposes the prolapsing mucosa to a high trans-mural pressure gradient which may lead to rupture of submucosal blood vessels with subsequent sloughing and ulceration of the mucosa.

Constipation

Most patients with constipation will be improved by an increased intake of dietary fibre. A proportion of patients are, however, made worse by this regimen. They complain of profound difficulty with rectal evacuation. Balloon expulsion studies [19] have suggested there is overactivity of the puborectalis and external anal sphincter muscles on attempted voiding. Defaecography in such patients [6] has demonstrated abnormal overactivity of the puborectalis and external anal sphincter on attempted voiding (Figure 4). This abnormality results in reduced widening of the ano-rectal angle on attempted voiding. Recent investigations have shown this abnormality to be equally distributed in patients with normal and slow transit constipation (unpublished observations). This finding suggests that an abnormality of the function of the pelvic

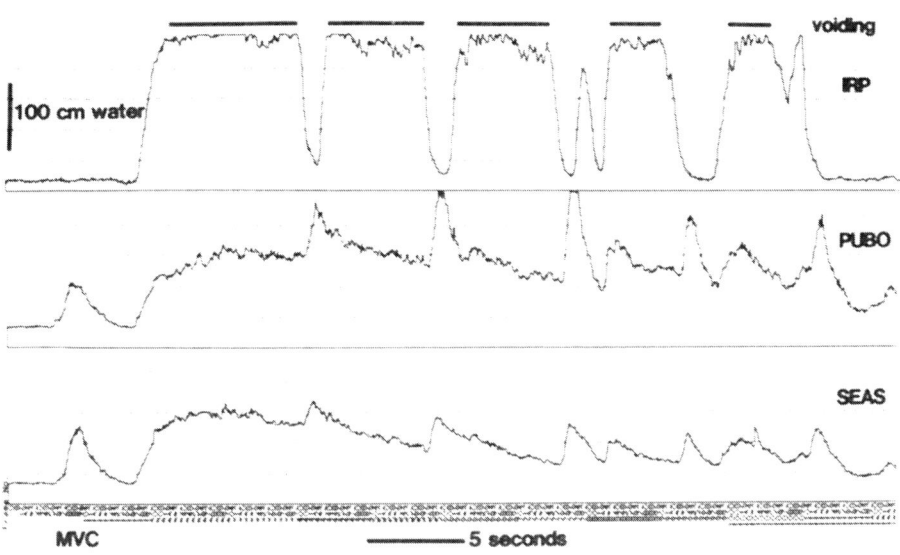

Figure 4. Intra-rectal pressure and sphincter EMG activity from a patient with constipation. Straining results in recruitment of sphincter EMG activity (Same key as in Figure 2).

floor musculature may be the underlying cause in most cases of idiopathic constipation.

Incontinence

In patients with idiopathic faecal incontinence there is perineal descent at rest with widening of the ano-rectal angle to 130° ± 3 (mean ± SEM cf. normal ano-rectal angle 92° ± 1.5 [12]. These changes are thought to result from neurogenic weakness of the pelvic floor and external anal sphincter muscles which may in turn result from excessive straining during defaecation. Defaecography has demonstrated overactivity of the sphincter muscles during voiding in incontinent patients with a history of straining at stool. Incontinent patients without a history of straining at stool had a normal pattern of sphincter inhibition during voiding. A high incidence of rectal intussusception (9 of 11 patients = 82%), was revealed in the incontinent patients. The incidence of intussusception was similar in the straining and non-straining groups and was clinically occult in six of the patients (unpublished observations). These findings suggest that abnormal function of the pelvic floor muscles may contribute to the aetiology of incontinence in patients who strain excessively at stool. However, the high incidence of intussusception in both groups implies that repeated dilation of the anal sphincters by a prolapse may be an important, yet hitherto under-estimated, factor in the aetiology of faecal incontinence.

40

Summary

Defaecography is at present performed only in a few proctological units. It is proving helpful in investigation of the aetiology of several ano-rectal conditions. It is possible, with such techniques, to diagnose abnormalities that are not clinically apparent. It therefore has a role in the investigation of patients with persistent, functional, ano-rectal symptoms where clinical investigation may be normal. Such cases include the solitary rectal ulcer syndrome, suspected rectal prolapse, and patients with symptoms of difficult, or incomplete, rectal evacuation.

References

1. Fry IK, Griffiths JD, Smart PLG. 1966. Some observations on the movement of the pelvic floor and rectum with special reference to rectal prolapse. Br J Surg 53: 784–787.
2. Broden B, Shellman B. 1968. Procidentia of the rectum studied with cineradiography: a contribution to the discussion of causative mechanism. Colon Rectum 11: 330–347.
3. Phillips SF, Edwards DAW. 1965. Some aspects of anal continence and defaecation. Gut 6: 396–405.
4. Kerremans R. 1969. Morphological and physiological aspects of anal continence and defaecation. Brussels; Editions Arscia.
5. Mahieu P, Pringot J, Bodart P. 1984. Defaecography: 1. Description of a new procedure and results in normal patients. Gastrointestinal Radiology 9: 247–251.
6. Womack NR, Williams NS, Holmfield JHM, Morrison JFB, Simpkins KC. 1985. New method for dynamic assessment of ano-rectal function in constipation. Br J Surg 72: 994–998.
7. Preston DM, Lennard-Jones JE, Thomas BM. 1984. The balloon proctogram. Br J Surg 71: 29–32.
8. Bartram CI, Mahieu PHG. 1985. Radiology of the pelvic floor. In: Henry MM, Swash M, (eds) Coloproctology and the pelvic floor: pathophysiology and management. London: Butterworths: 151–186.
9. Parks AG, Forter N, Melzak J. 1962. Experimental study of the reflex mechanism controlling the muscles of the pelvic floor. Colon Rectum 5: 407–414.
10. Womack NR, Morrison JFB, Williams NS. 1985. Impaired recruitment of the pelvic floor musculature by intra-abdominal pressure in faecal incontinence. Gut: 26–31.
11. Parks AG. 1975. Ano-rectal incontinence. Proc R Soc Med 68: 681–690.
12. Mahieu P, Pringot J, Bodart P. 1984. Defaecography 2.: Contribution to the diagnosis of defaecation disorders. Gastrointestinal Radiology 9: 253—261.
13. Madigan MR, Morson BC. 1969. Solitary ulcer of the rectum. Gut 10: 871–881.
14. Rutter KRP, Riddell RH. 1975. The solitary ulcer syndrome of the rectum. Clin Gastroenterol 4: 505–530.
15. Mahieu P, Pringot J, Vanheuverzwijn, Goncette L. 1981. Les prolapses du rectum. Acta Gastroent Belg 44: 502–512.
16. Rutter KRP. 1974. Electromyographic changes in certain pelvic floor abnormalities. Proc R Soc Med 67: 53–56.
17. Womack NR, Holmfield JHM, Morrison JFB, Williams NS. 1986. Ano-rectal function in the solitary rectal ulcer syndrome (SRUS). Br J Surg (in press).
18. Du Boulay C, Fairbrother J, Isaacson PG. 1983. Mucosal prolapse syndrome – a unifying concept for solitary ulcer syndrome and related disorders. J Clin Pathol 36: 1264–1268.
19. Preston DM, Lennard-Jones JE. 1985. Anismus in chronic constipation. Dig Dis Sci 30: 413–418.

1.4 Ano-rectal sensation

N.J. McC MORTENSEN & A.M. ROE

Introduction

Whilst the bulk of published work on disordered defaecation has concentrated on the motor function of the anal sphincter [1, 2], ano-rectal sensation may also play a crucial role in the preservation of continence, but there are surprisingly few published data on the subject.

Innervation

The anal canal above the anal valves is derived from endodermal cloaca, and is supplied by autonomic nerves. Below this level the anal canal arises from ectodermal proctoderm, and here it is supplied by spinal nerves – the inferior rectal nerve, a branch of the pudendal nerve arising from the anterior primary rami of the second, third and fourth spinal nerves, and by direct branches of motor roots S3 & S4 lying on the upper surface of the pelvic floor.

Careful histological studies have demonstrated various types of nerve endings in the anal canal epithelium in man [3]. Duthie and Gairns [4] found free intra-epithelial and organised nerve endings in profusion around the anal valves, but no endings in the mucosa of the rectum (Figure 1).

Normal sensation

Duthie and Gairns [4] were also able to show that by qualitative testing the anal canal is sensitive to pain, heat and cold, touch and movement. Pain could be felt as far as 1.5 cm above the anal valves, and this corresponds with clinical experience in injecting or rubber band ligation of haemorrhoids. An incorrectly placed band can give rise to intense pain even 2 cm from the dentate line in some subjects.

42

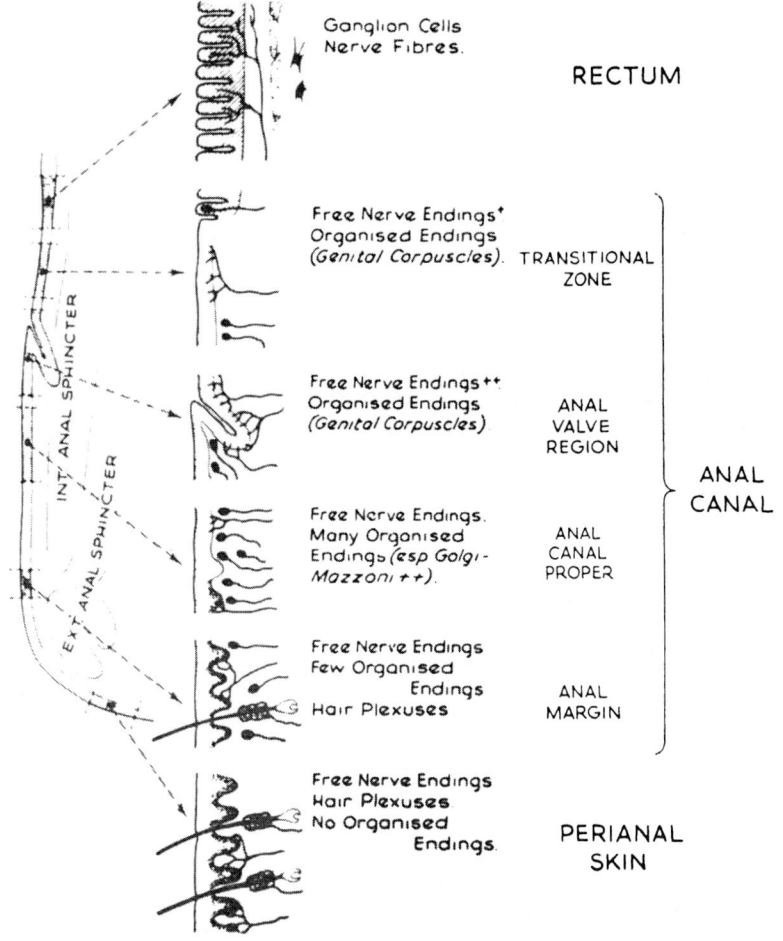

Figure 1. Sensory nerve endings in the anal canal (after Duthie and Gairns [4]).

The patients awareness of rectal distension is characterised by a distinct sensation localised to the rectum or sacral area. The receptors responsible for this sensation probably do not reside in the rectum itself, since patients with low rectal carcinoma treated by resection of the rectum and a colo-anal anastomosis preserve the normal filling sensations and recto-anal inhibitory reflex [5], and stretch receptors have been identified in the levator muscles [6]. A more precise perception of the nature of rectal contents could be a function of intra-rectal pressure [7] flatus giving rise to lower pressures than solid stool.

Duthie and Bennett [8] have suggested that this discrimination between solid, liquid, and gas is achieved by sensory receptors in the anal canal. When intra-rectal pressure rises, the upper anal canal opens allowing the rectal contents to be sampled. Just how important this sensory zone is for continence, however, remains controversial. Goligher [9] found that patients treated by colo-anal anastomosis could not distinguish between flatus and faeces, perhaps as a result of excision of the crucial sensory zone. Read and Read [10], however, using a saline continence test could find no effect when the anal canal was anaesthetised with lignocaine and concluded that sensation does not play a crucial role in normal continence.

Abnormal sensation

In the incontinent patient it may be difficult to demonstrate whether a sensory deficit compounds the problems produced by a motor weakness in the sphincters. Certainly patients with ano-rectal incontinence often report that they have no sense of an impending or completed episode of incontinence, and cannot distinguish between gas or liquid in the anal canal. Read and Abouzekry [11] in studying the reasons for faecal incontinence in elderly patients with faecal impaction found that light touch and pain sensation in the anal canal and peri-anal region were normal in control subjects. In contrast, peri-anal sensation was absent or impaired in 74% of impacted patients, whilst anal canal sensation was absent or impaired in 77%. Gunterberg [12] studied patients after major resections of the sacrum with bilateral or unilateral sacrifice of sacral nerves. Those with a bilateral loss had impaired discrimination between different qualities of rectal contents passing through the anal canal, and impaired sensation of rectal distension. Total one sided denervation resulted in a unilaterally deficient anal canal sensation but no disturbance of sphincter function.

Anal sensation has also been studied by observing somatosensory evoked potentials after an anal stimulus. In infants over 4 months old anal somatosensory evoked potentials can be recorded, but in one study were absent in one child with meningo-myelocele but present in two following pull-through operations for rectal atresia and imperforate anus [13]. Normal subjects are able to prevent accidental faecal leakage because they can perceive the levels of rectal distension which would usually cause relaxation of the internal anal sphincter and conciously contract the external anal sphincter to prevent incontinence. Read and Abouzekry have also shown [11] that in patients with faecal impaction for example, rectal sensation is blunted and external sphincter contraction in response to rectal distension occurred at higher distending volumes than controls. In addition, anal sphincter relaxation occurred at lower levels of rectal distension. Similar abnormalities of rectal sensation have been suggested in the incontinence of diabetics, myelomeningocele patients and children with encopresis [14, 15].

Measuring anal canal sensation

Although Duthie and Gairns [4] were able to demonstrate that it is possible to test for anal sensation like cutaneous sensation, this is a rather impractical and subjective assessment. We have therefore developed a technique [16] based on the principle of mucosal electrosensitivity to measure anal sensation described and first used in clinical urology by Kieswetter [17] and Powell [18].

A catheter was constructed with two platinum electrodes placed 1 cm apart towards the tip of a 10 Fr gauge Dover catheter graduated in cm. Copper wires connected to these electrodes were attached to a constant current generator supplying square wave stimuli of 100 μsec duration at 5 pulses per second. There is an inbuilt compensation for the impedance of a tissue under study, enabling the observer to reliably determine that the probe is in contact with the anal mucosa.

Patients were examined in the left lateral position and the functional length of the anal canal determined using a water filled microballoon manometric system. The electrosensitivity probe was lubricated with a conductive mixture of saline and gel and placed in the anal canal. The current across the electrodes was then increased incrementally until a threshold sensation was reported by the patient, usually as a burning or tingling sensation, and recordings made at three levels within the anal canal (Figure 2).

Using this technique we have studied 97 patients – 20 control subjects, 17 with incontinence, 10 with fissure in ano, 28 with haemorrhoids and 22 with slow transit constipation. In normal control subjects the sensory threshold varied from 2 to 7.3 mA being most acute in the middle site corresponding to the position of the anal valves where the sensory nerve endings are concentrated (Figure 3). There were no significant differences in sensory thresholds in normal subjects between the sexes (5 men, 15 women) or with increasing age (over or under 60 years). The results of anal mucosal sensory threshold measurements are shown in Table 1: the higher the figure the less sensitive the mucosa.

Patients with incontinence had a shorter functional sphincter than controls, 2.5 (0–3.5) cm versus 3.25 cm (3.0–4.0) cm, ($p<0.02$). Therefore measurements were made at two sites only in the upper and lower sphincter.

These results confirm that patients with idiopathic faecal incontinence have a sensory deficit (Figure 4). In haemorrhoid patients a low sensitivity in the upper anal canal might be explained by the displacement of insensitive rectal mucosa into the upper anal canal (Figure 5). Anal sensation was not impaired in slow transit constipation patients, but not surprisingly those with a fissure in ano were very sensitive.

So we have been able to demonstrate objective differences in anal canal sensation in various ano-rectal disorders. Clearly an elaborate and sophisti-

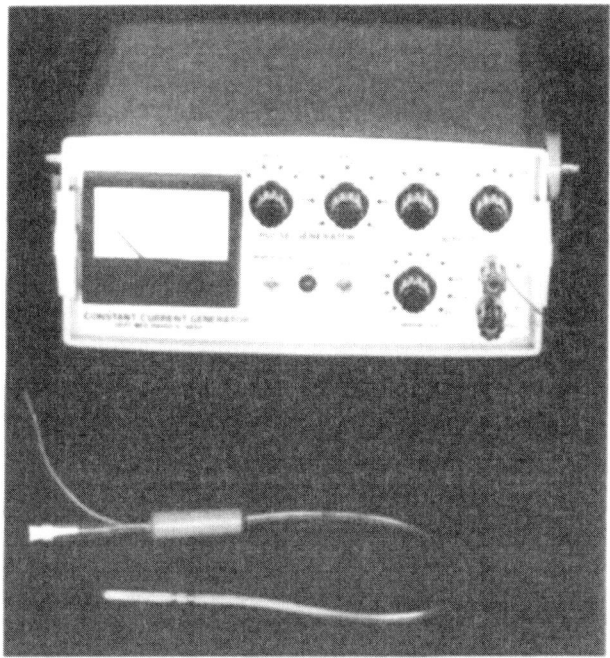

Figure 2. The electrosensitivity probe and constant current generator.

cated sensory system is present but there is no clear evidence to show how this might work. In normal skin the appreciation of 'wetness' is a blended sensory experience that depends on the activation of a mixture of sensory channels that evoke mechanical and thermal sensations [19]. The time course and rate of change of cutaneous thermal stimuli determine the perception of blended

Table 1. Comparison of anal mucosal sensory threshold under different pathological conditions with normal controls.

	Anal mucosal sensory threshold in mA: medians and ranges		
	Lower	Middle	Upper
Controls	4.8 (3.0–7.0)	4.2 (2.0–6.0)	5.7 (3.3–7.3)
Incontinent[++]	8. (4.3–11.0)[a]	–	8.7 (6.0–23.0)[a]
Haemorrhoids	5.9 (1.7–10.0)	6.3 (1.3–16.7)[b]	9.8 (4.0–20.0)[c]
Fissure	2.0 (1.3–4.0)[a]	3.2 (1.3–5.0)	4.5 (3.0–12.0)
Slow transit constipation	5.0 (2.0–7.0)	4.8 (2.6–8.7)	6.2 (3.0–11.0)

[++] Measurements at two sites only because of short sphincter length. [a] $p<0.002$ versus controls; [b] $p<0.01$ versus controls; [c] $p<0.0001$ versus controls. Mann Whitney U Test.

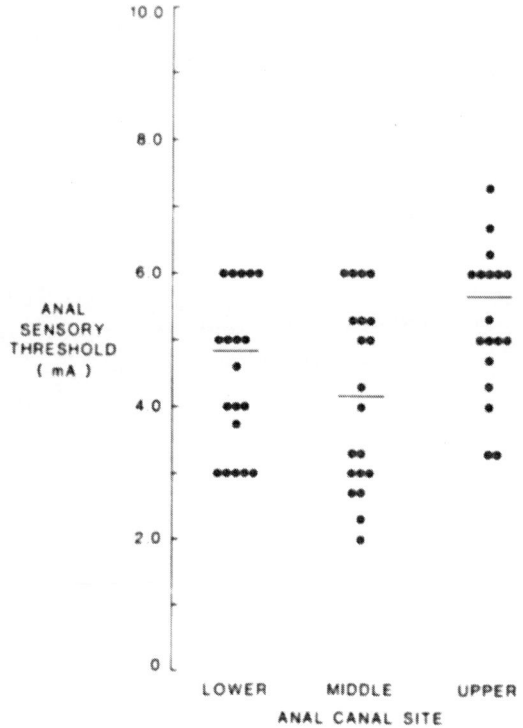

Figure 3. Anal sensation in normal subjects. Sensation is most acute in the middle site corresponding to the anal valves.

sensations [20] and it is possible that the sensory arc of the sampling reflex
works in this way.

It is important to distinguish between conscious appreciation of rectal filling
and those unconscious recto-anal responses to rectal filling and anal canal
contents which nevertheless require sensory receptors for functioning reflexes. The most widely known of these is the recto-anal inhibitory reflex,
usually absent in patients with Hirschsprung's disease.

Rectal sensation

The simplest method for measuring rectal sensation is to place a balloon in the
rectum and inflate it with increasing volumes of air [21]. The volume at which
the first sensation is appreciated can be recorded, and with increasing volumes
of air the maximum tolerable volume can be reached. Some authors advocate

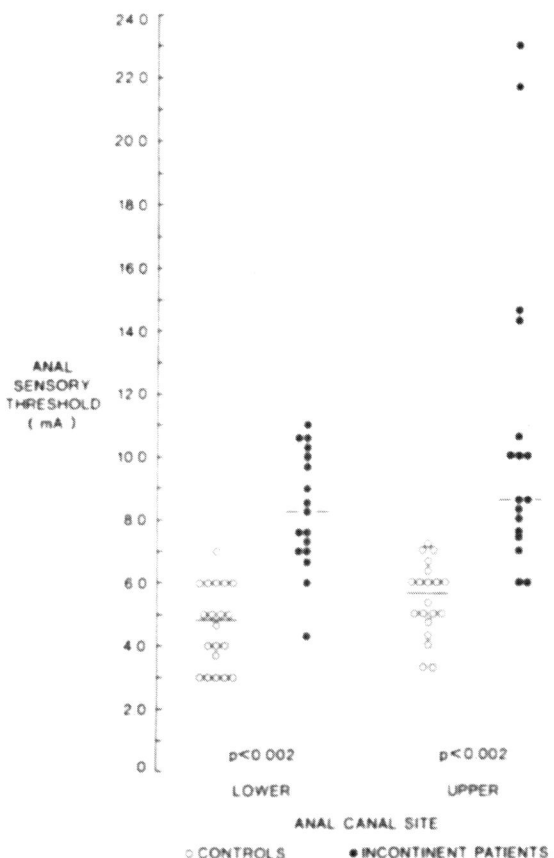

Figure 4. Anal sensation in idiopathic faecal incontinence showing higher sensory thresholds throughout the anal canal ○ controls, ● incontinent patients.

the use of water as the distending agent since a correction for pressure and temperature is then not necessary.

A more sophisticated method of measurement involves the use of a constant infusion of fluid into a rectal balloon. The rectum acts as a dynamic reservoir for faeces, and like the urinary bladder this depends on the functional capacity of the rectum and its contractile properties [22], as well as perception of filling. Preston et al. [23] described such a method of measuring rectal pressure and volume in constipated patients, and called, by analogy with the cystometrogram, a proctometrogram. Not only can rectal sensation be recorded but the pressures at which sensation are noted can be measured [24]. Patients with constipation [23, 25], inflammatory bowel disease [26] and following low anterior resection have been studied in this way.

48

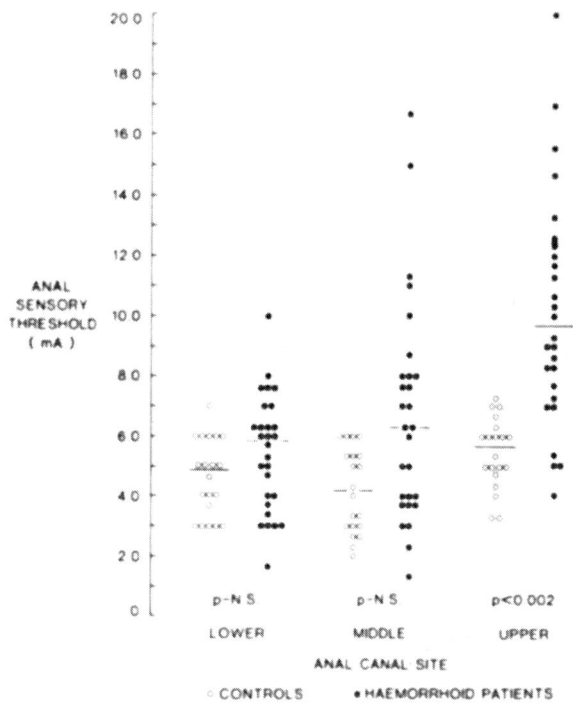

Figure 5. Anal sensation in patients with haemorrhoids. The mucosa is less sensitive in the middle and upper anal canal ○ controls, ● haemorrhoid patients.

Recto-anal responses

Distension of the rectum with a balloon normally induces a brief increase in anal pressure, caused by contraction of the external sphincter, and a decrease in anal pressure caused by relaxation of the internal sphincter [28, 29]. Although abnormalities of this response could be due to defects anywhere along the afferent or efferent parts of the reflex, it is still a useful method of assessing rectal sensation.

With a balloon in the rectum and a manometric catheter in the anal canal measuring the maximum resting pressure, the rectal ampulla is distended by inflating the balloon with air in increments of 10 ml, distension being maintained for 60 seconds. The balloon is then deflated and after a rest period refilled with the original volume plus 10 ml for a further 60 seconds. Rectal volumes are increased in this way until anal tone fails to recover with the balloon inflated.

Acknowledgements

Thanks to the British Journal of Surgery for permission to publish Figures 1, 3, 4 and 5.

References

1. Neill ME, Swash M. 1980. Increased motor unit fibre density in the external anal sphincter in ano-rectal incontinence: a single fibre EMG study. J Neurol Neurosurg Psych 43: 343–347.
2. Kiff ES, Swash M. 1984. Slowed conduction in the pudendal nerves in idiopathic (neurogenic) faecal incontinence. Br J Surg 71: 614–616.
3. Kantner M. 1957. Neue morphologische Ergebnisse Über die peripherischen Nervenaus-breitungen und ihre Deutung. Acta Anat 31: 397–425.
4. Duthie HL, Gairns FW. 1960. Sensory nerve endings and sensation in the anal region of man. Br. J Surg 47: 584–594.
5. Lane RHS, Parks AG. 1977. Function of the anal sphincters following colo-anal anastomoses. Br J Surg 64: 596–599.
6. Williams NS, Price R, Johnston D. 1980. The long term effects of sphincter preserving operations for rectal carcinoma on function of anal sphincter in man. Br J Surg 67: 203–208.
7. Goligher JC, Hughes ESR. 1951. Sensibility of the rectum and colon: its role in the mechanism of anal continence. Lancet i: 543–548.
8. Duthie HL, Bennett RC. 1963. The relation of sensation in the anal canal to the functional anal sphincter: a possible factor in anal continence. Gut 4: 179–182.
9. Goligher JC. 1951. The functional results after sphincter saving resections of the rectum. Ann Roy Coll Surg Engl 8: 421–439.
10. Read MG, Read NW. 1982. The role of ano-rectal sensation in preserving continence. Gut 23: 345–347.
11. Read NW, Abouzekry L. 1986. Why do patients with faecal impaction have faecal inconti-nence? Gut 27: 283–287.
12. Gunterberg B, Kewenter J, Petersen I, Stener B. 1976. Ano-rectal function after major resections of the sacrum with bilateral or unilateral sacrifice of sacral nerves. Br J Surg 63: 546–54.
13. Sedgewick EM. 1982. Clinical application of the spinal and cortical somatosensory evoked potentials. Amsterdam: Excerpta Medica: 207–214.
14. Wald A, Tununguntla AK. 1984. Ano-rectal sensation dysfunction in faecal incontinence and diabetes mellitus. N Engl J Med 310: 1282–1287.
15. Meunier P, Mollard P, Marechal J-M. 1976. Physiology of megarectum: the association of megarectum with encopresis. Gut 17: 224–227.
16. Roe AM, Bartolo DCC, Mortensen NJMcC. 1986. A new method for assessment of anal sensation in various ano-rectal disorders. Br J Surg 73: 310–312.
17. Kieswetter H. 1977. Mucosal sensory threshold of urinary bladder and urethra measured electrically. Urologia Internationalis 32: 437–448.
18. Powell PH, Feneley RCL. 1980. The role of urethral sensation in clinical urology. Br J Urol 52: 539–541.
19. Schmidt RF, ed. 1981. Fundamentals of sensory physiology. Springer-Verlag, New York-Heidelberg-Berlin.
20. Sinclair D. 1981. Mechanisms of cutaneous sensation. Oxford University Press, Oxford.

21. Farthing MJG, Lennard-Jones JE. 1978. Sensibility of the rectum to distension and the ano-rectal distension reflex in ulcerative colitis. Gut 19: 64–69.
22. Arhan P, Fanerdin C, Persoz B, Devroede G, Dubois F, Dornic C, Pellerin D. 1976. Relationship between viscoelastic properties of the rectum and anal pressure in man. J Appl Physiol 41: 677–682.
23. Preston DM, Barnes PRH, Lennard-Jones JE. 1983. Proctometrogram: does it have a role in the evaluation of adults with chronic constipation? Gut 24: A1010–1011.
24. Varma JS, Smith AN. 1986. Reproducibility of the proctometrogram. Gut 27: 288–292.
25. Roe AM, Mortensen NJMcC. 1985. Why do patients with slow transit constipation have no postprandial defaecation response? Br J Surg 72: S141.
26. Keighley MRB, Buchmann P, Lee RJ. 1982. Assessment of ano-rectal function in selection of patients for ileo-rectal anastomosis in Crohn's colitis. Gut 23: 102–107.
27. Suzuki H, Matsumoto K, Amano S, Fujioka M, Honsumi M. 1980. Ano-rectal pressure and rectal compliance after low anterior resection. Br J Surg 67: 655–657.
28. Schuster MM, Hendrix TR, Mendellof AL. 1963. The internal sphincter response. Manometric studies on its normal physiology, normal pathways, and alteration in bowel disease. J Clin Invest 42: 196–207.
29. Read MG, Read NW, Barber DC, Duthie HK. 1982. Effect of loperamide on anal sphincter function in patients complaining of chronic diarrhoea with faecal incontinence and urgency. Dig Dis Sci 27: 807–814.

1.5 Colonic motility

A.J.P.M. SMOUT

Introduction

The three main functions of the colon, the absorption of sodium and water, the intraluminal metabolism of undigested nutrients by bacteria and the temporary storage and controlled evacuation of faeces, are closely interrelated. The motor activity of the colon is of primary importance for the last mentioned function, but indirectly influences the other functions as well. Disturbances of colonic motility may lead to constipation or diarrhoea, both of which may be involved in the pathogenesis of faecal incontinence. Unfortunately, our knowledge of human colonic motility in health and disease is still rather limited and many of our concepts are not based on consistent results of appropriate studies.

In this chapter the available information on the physiology of colonic motility will be summarised. The most important abnormalities of colonic motility presently thought to be involved in the pathogenesis of constipation and diarrhoea will be indicated.

Methods used in in-vivo studies of colonic motility

Since the beginning of this century *radiographic techniques* have been used to study the motility of the colon filled with a barium or bismuth salt suspension [1–8]. The advantage of this method is that it provides information on colonic contractile activity at various sites at the same time, as well as information on the effects of these contractions on the colonic contents. In fact, our present knowledge of the gross motility patterns of the colon (animal or human) still depends largely upon information gathered in fluoroscopic studies performed many years ago. The most important disadvantages of the method are the exposure to ionising radiation and the hardly quantifiable nature of the observations.

Intraluminal pressure measurement, either with fluid or air-filled balloons, with open-tip perfused catheters or with miniature strain-gauge transducers has frequently been used to study colonic motility, especially in man. With this method prolonged recordings can be made, quantitative data can be obtained. The major problem is that the relations between contractions of the colonic wall and intraluminal pressure changes are inconsistent [4].

Electromyography of colonic smooth muscle can be performed via two ways of approach, from the serosal side (mostly in laboratory animals such as the cat and the dog), or from the luminal side (mostly in man). The electrodes can be monopolar or bipolar, the latter being more popular. Intraluminal electrodes may either be allowed to float freely in the colonic lumen [9, 10], or be attached to the mucosa by means of clipping or suction [11, 12]. Even with an attached type of electrode the investigator is not always sure whether the electrode is still in contact with the mucosa, since the nature of the colonic myoelectrical signal in man often does not allow its differentiation from noise (vide infra).

Extraluminal force measurement with the aid of implanted strain gauge transducers is a technique that provides meaningful and quantifiable data, but the use of these transducers is restricted to laboratory animals.

Radionuclide techniques can be used to study colonic transit. The radio-isotope labeled material can be introduced into the colon by consumption by mouth [5] or through a tube that traverses the small intestine [13].

Radio-opaque markers, ingested by mouth, are used in many clinics to study colonic transit in constipated patients. Serial x-rays of the abdomen can be made to study the day-to-day changes in distribution of the markers over the colon [14], or the faeces can be x-rayed.

Patterns of colonic motility

Radiographic studies in man and in laboratory animals have suggested that, as far as gross motility patterns are concerned, the colon can be divided into three parts [1, 2, 6, 7], in the first part, consisting of the coecum, the ascending colon and the proximal part of the transverse colon, retrograde ('antiperistaltic') contractions occur. In cats and dogs the fundamental frequency of these contractions is 5–6/min. In man frequencies of 5–6/min are also predominant, but lower and higher frequencies are present as well.

In the second part of the colon, consisting of the distal transverse colon, the descending colon and the sigmoid colon, 'segmenting' contractions predominate. These variably deep, circular contractions are either stationary or are propagated orally or aborally over short distances. In the cat their maximum frequency is slightly higher than in the first and third part of the colon. In man various contractile frequencies have been described. These segmenting con-

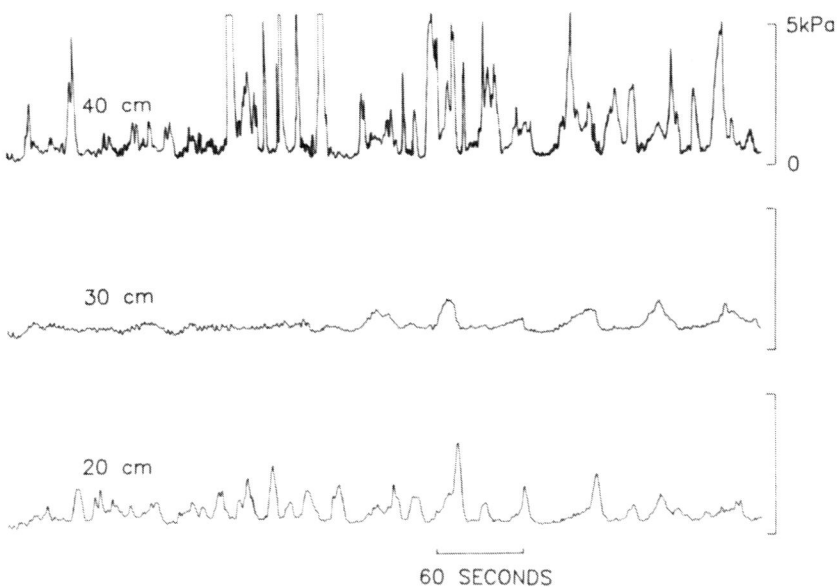

Figure 1. Intraluminal pressure recordings simultaneously obtained from three adjacent sites in the human colon. The signals recorded from these three sites show little if any correlation.

tractions are responsible for the haustrated appearance of the colon. It has been demonstrated that the position of the haustral folds is not fixed; haustra constantly disappear and reform at different locations [6].

The third part, consisting of the rectum and possibly of the distal part of the sigmoid colon, serves as a reservoir. In this part of the colon the contractions are said to be predominantly caudad moving. In cats and dogs their fundamental frequency is 5–6/min. In man, no specific contraction frequency prevails, but the existence of two frequency bands has been described: a band of 2–4/min and a band of 6–12/min. As illustrated in Figure 1, the contractions in this part of the human colon, as studied with intraluminal pressure recording, are extremely variable from minute to minute and from one recording site to another [15].

So-called mass movements have been observed in all parts of the colon [1–3, 5, 7]. These movements are brought about by strong aborally propagating contractions of long segments of colon. They occur infrequently (a few times per day?), mostly shortly after eating. The mass contractions are preceded by temporary disappearance of haustral (segmenting) contractions. Mass movements swiftly transport faeces towards the distal colon and rectum and may initiate the process of defaecation.

The results of several studies are consistent with the concept that the motility of the sigmoid forms a barrier on the transit of faeces. In this concept hyperactivity leads to constipation and hypoactivity contributes to diarrhoea [16–18]. However, the pathophysiology of constipation is not covered by this single mechanism, since many constipated patients have normal or diminished sigmoid motility [19, 20].

Recto-anal motility

Rectal distension (by faeces or by balloon inflation) evokes the so-called recto-anal inhibition reflex resulting in unvoluntary relaxation of the internal anal sphincter, which is composed of smooth muscle. Rectal distension also gives rise to sensations that warn the subject that defaecation is imminent. It is not yet clear where the receptors involved in these sensations are located. Receptors in the proximal anal canal allow the subject to discriminate between a solid, fluid or gaseous nature of the rectal contents.

When defaecation has to be postponed, the striated external anal sphincter and the musculature of the pelvic floor are contracted. Among the pelvic floor muscles the U-shaped puborectalis muscle forms an important distinct structure that brings about the angle between the longitudinal axes of rectum and anal canal. When defaecation is permitted, the pelvic floor and the external anal sphincter are relaxed, the recto-anal angle straightens.

The recto-anal mechanisms involved in maintenance of continence and in the process of defaecation will be discussed in greater detail in other chapters of this book. At this place it suffices to emphasize the important role in normal defaecation played by these recto-anal mechanisms. It becomes increasingly clear that in a substantial proportion of the patients suffering from severe constipation diminished or absent relaxation of pelvic floor muscles and the external anal sphincter is responsible for their inability to defaecate [20, 21]. This form of constipation is called outlet obstruction.

Normal defaecation is further accomplished by increasing the intra-abdominal pressure, by rectal contractions, and possibly also by ongoing mass movements, since it has been shown that some individuals empty their entire left colon in defaecation [22].

Myogenic control of colonic motility

From the stomach and the small bowel periodical potential variations, which are not directly contraction-related, can be recorded. These omnipresent waves are often referred to as slow waves or Electrical Control Activity (ECA) [23]. Upper digestive tract ECA is highly regular and propagates in aboral direction.

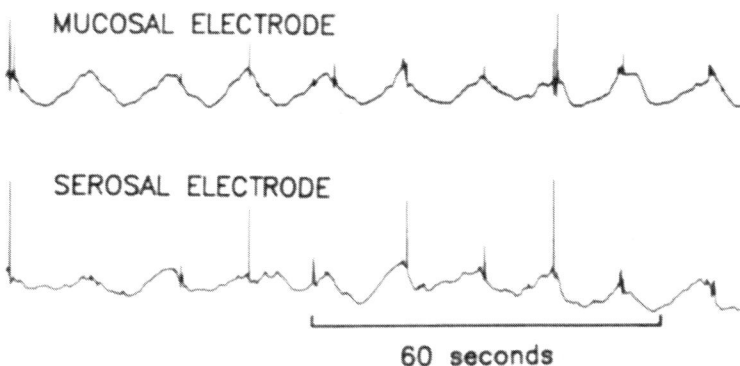

Figure 2. Myoelectrical activities of the colon in an anaesthetised dog. The upper trace shows the signal recorded from a bipolar intraluminal needle electrode held against the mucosa. The lower trace shows the signal simultaneously recorded from a bipolar needle electrode sutured to the serosal surface of the colon, directly opposite the mucosal electrode. Both signals show regular ECA with a frequency of about 5/min. Spike activity (ERA) is present in several of the ECA cycles.

A second type of electrical activity, called spike activity or Electrical Response Activity (ERA) occurs intermittently, superimposed upon the slow wave. When ERA occurs, a contraction follows. In the upper parts of the digestive tract ECA thus controls time, site and propagation of phasic contractions.

In the colon of the cat and the dog regular slow wave activity (ECA) can also be observed (Figure 2). The frequeny of the ECA in these species rises from 4.5/min in the proximal part to 6.0/min in the most distal part [24]. These frequencies correspond nicely to the contractile frequencies observed in the cat colon [1, 2]. The effect of sectioning of the cat colon into rings is greatest in the most proximal parts of the colon where the ECA frequency undergoes the greatest drop [24]. This low intrinsic ECA frequency in the proximal colon is considered to give rise to predominantly oral propagation of the ECA, which is in accordance with the predominantly antiperistaltic contraction waves observed in this part of the cat colon [1, 2].

There is evidence that indicates that the ECA in the colon of the cat is generated in the circular muscle layer, and not in the longitudinal layer [25]. In the canine colon the longitudinal muscle layer has been shown to generate a distinct type of oscillatory electrical activity.

In the human colon in-situ ECA is much more irregular than in the canine and feline colon (Figure 3). According to some investigators it is even absent during up to 80% of time [11, 12]. These findings may be explained by recent observations on the electrical activity of the human colon in vitro [26, 27]. Although spontaneous electrical oscillation (ECA) was continuously present

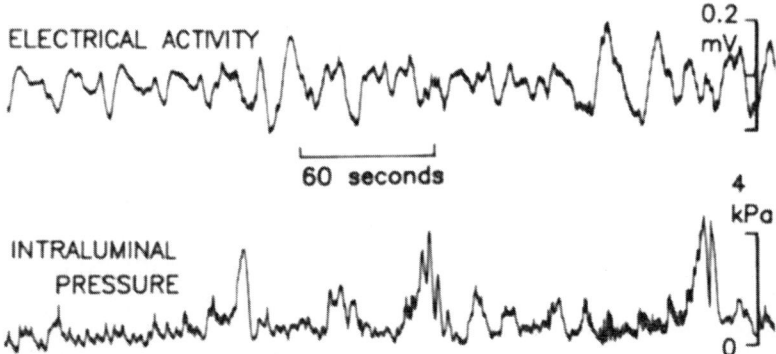

Figure 3. Myoelectrical (upper trace) and intraluminal pressure (lower trace) signals simultaneously recorded from the sigmoid colon in man. The myoelectrical signal, recorded with a bipolar needle electrode held against the mucosa by means of suction, shows oscillations of variable frequency and amplitude.

in most circular muscle strips of human colon, the amplitude of this activity was low (lower than in the dog) and the frequency of the oscillations varied dramatically within a range from 4.5 to 60 cycles/min. Contractile activity accompanied oscillatory activity alone as well as oscillation with superimposed spikes. Contractions associated with ECA frequencies above 12 cycles/min were found to show summation. In the longitudinal muscle layer bursts of oscillations with a frequency in a relatively narrow range from 24 to 36 cycles/min were observed. Both the oscillations and the superimposed spiking activity were related to fused contractions.

Unlike gastric and small intestinal ECA, human colonic ECA has been shown to depend strongly upon stretch and activation by neurotransmitters and hormones [26].

In patients with the Irritable Bowel Syndrome of either the constipation-predominant or the diarrhoea-predominant type an increased incidence of rectosigmoid slow wave activity with a frequency of about 3/min, has been reported [11, 28].

In the colon of man and other species not only short spike bursts (SSB) or 'discrete ERA' (DERA) can occur, but also prolonged spike bursts, also called 'long spike bursts' (LSB), or 'continuous ERA' (CERA), are observed (Figure 4). The latter extend over several slow waves and are accompanied by a prolonged contraction.

In accordance with earlier studies on sigmoid motor activity in patients with the Irritable Bowel Syndrome, diminished spike activity was found in patients with predominant diarrhoea and increased spike activity in patients with predominant constipation [11, 29].

A third type of contraction-related electrical activity observed in the human

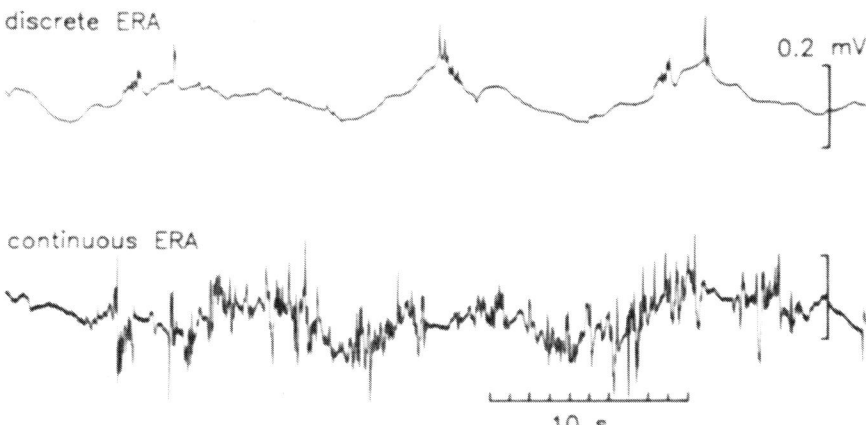

Figure 4. Two types of contraction-related electrical activity observed in the colon. Discrete ERA is limited to a segment of th ECA cycle, continuous ERA (long spike burst) spans several ECA cycles. Anaesthetised dog, bipolar serosal electrodes.

colon consists of sinusoidal oscillations with a frequency of 25–40 cycles/min that are also accompanied by contractions of long duration. This type of activity has been called 'contractile electrical complex' (CEC) [30]. It seems possible that these are identical to the electrical oscillations observed in in-vitro preparations of the longitudinal muscle layer [26, 27]. Furthermore, although this has not yet been described in the human colon in-situ, prolonged contractions can apparently be induced by SBBs (DERA) when the frequency of the slow waves upon which they are superimposed is above 12 cycles/min [26].

It must be concluded that the relatively simple concepts of myogenic control of gastric and small intestinal motility are not applicable to the human colon. It is doubtful whether the term 'Electrical Control Activity' is appropriate to designate the oscillatory potentials recorded from colonic smooth muscle in man. The pathophysiological significance of the reported slow wave abnormalities in the Irritable Bowel Syndrome is unclear.

Neurogenic control of colonic motility

The neurogenic control of colonic motility involves extrinsic and intrinsic neuronal systems. The extrinsic system consists of parasympathetic neurons, reaching the colon through the vagus and pelvic nerves, and sympathetic neurons with cell bodies in the superior and inferior mesenteric ganglia, reaching the colon through perivascular plexuses. The intrinsic neurons are grouped in a number of intramural plexuses, the most extensive of which is the plexus of Auerbach. The circuitry of the intrinsic colonic nerves has not yet been elucidated to the full. Apart from excitatory cholinergic and inhibitory adrenergic nerves, excitatory noncholinergic and inhibitory nonadrenergic nerves are present in the colon. Their mediators are unknown (VIP, ATP?).

The net effect of the neural control mechanism seems to be that of an inhibition of motility. After spinal cord transsection colonic motility is increased, but the postprandial motility increase (gastrocolonic response) is blunted [31].

In patients with severe idiopathic constipation morphological abnormalities of the myenteric plexus have been found [32]. Although it is tempting to ascribe the constipation of these patients to the neuronal abnormalities, such a causal relation has not been proven beyond doubt. The neuronal changes might result from chronic use of laxatives or from chronic stretch of the colonic wall caused by the constipation.

There is no doubt that stress of several types has considerable effects on colonic motility, both in health and disease [33–35]. The effect of stress on colonic motility can be decreased by tranquilizers [35].

Hormonal control of colonic motility

Many of the presently known gastrointestinal hormones have effects on colonic motility. It is far from certain, however, that all the reported effects are of physiological significance. Some substances known as hormones may also be involved in neuroneuronal transmission or affect colonic motility through a paracrine mechanism (e.g., VIP, somatostatin, enkephalin). Physiological doses of gastrin and cholecystokinin increase colonic motility in man. The postprandial release of these hormones by the proximal gut seems to play a role in the gastrocolonic response, but other hormonal as well as neuronal mechanisms also appear to be involved.

In patients with the Irritable Bowel Syndrome the colonic motor and spike activity response to a meal has been found to be increased or prolonged [17, 36]. This finding could not be corroborated by another group of investigators [37].

Summary and conclusions

As far as its motility is concerned, the colon undoubtedly is the most obscure part of the human alimentary canal. Its contractile activity is hardly quantifiable, its electrical slow waves do not really deserve the predicate 'control activity' and only scattered information on the neuronal and hormonal control of its motor activity is available.

Nevertheless, it is clear that normal colonic motility is essential for the preservation of well-being and that disturbances of colonic motility can lead to disabling symptoms. Recent studies have shed more light on some important aspects of normal colonic motor function. Some of the pathophysiological mechanisms that play a role in such common disorders as constipation and the irritable bowel syndrome have been clarified.

However, a strong need for more (patho)physiological information on colonic motility is felt by both basic scientists and clinicians. Given the time-varying and stimulus-sensitive nature of colonic motility, the employment of minimally invasive techniques that allow for prolonged observation must be considered indispensable in studies of colonic motility in health and disease.

References

1. Cannon WB. 1902. The movements of the intestines studied by means of the rontgen rays. Am J Physiol 6: 251–277.
2. Elliott TR, Barclay-Smith E. 1904 Antiperistalsis and other muscular activities of the colon. J Physiol (London) 31: 272–304.
3. Hertz Af, Newton A. 1913. The normal movements of the colon in man. J Physiol (London) 47: 57–65.
4. Deller DJ, Wangel AG. 1965. Intestinal motility in man. I. A study combining the use of intraluminal pressure recording and cineradiography. Gastroenterology 48: 45–57.
5. Holdstock DJ, Misiewicz JJ, Smith T, Rowlands EN. 1970. Propulsion (mass movements) in the human colon and its relationships to meals and somatic activity. Gut 11: 91–99.
6. Ritchie JA. 1971. Movement of segmental constrictions in the human colon. Gut 12: 350–355.
7. Ritchie JA. 1972. Mass peristalsis in the human colon after contact with oxyphenisatin. Gut 13: 211–219.
8. Ritchie JA, Adrian GM, Truelove SC. 1962. Motor activity of the sigmoid colon of humans. A combined study by intraluminal pressure recording and cineradiography. Gastroenterology 43: 642–648.
9. Fioramonti J, Bueno L, Frexinos J. 1980. Sonde endoluminale pour l'exploration électromyographique de la motricité colique chez l'homme. Gastroenterol Clin Biol 4: 546–550.
10. Schang JC, Devroede G. 1983. Fasting and postprandial myoelectric spiking activity in the human sigmoid colon. Gastroenterology 85: 1048–1053.
11. Snape WJ, Carlson GM, Cohen S. 1976. Colonic myoelectric activity in the irritable bowel syndrome. Gastroenterology 70: 326–330.
12. Taylor I, Duthie HL, Smallwood R, Linkens R. 1975. Large bowel myoelectrical activity in man. Gut 19: 808–814.
13. Krevsky B, Malmud LS, Somers MB, Siegel JA, Maurer AH, Fisher RS. 1986. Patterns of colonic transit in chronic idiopathic constipation (abstr). Gastroenterology 90: 1503.
14. Martelli H, Devroede G, Arhan P, Duguay C, Dornic C, Faverdin C. 1978. Some parameters of large bowel motility in normal man. Gastroenterology 75: 612–618.
15. Dinoso VP, Murthy SNS, Goldstein J, Rosner B. 1983. Basal motor activity of the distal colon: a reappraisal. Gastroenterology 85: 637–642.
16. Connell AM. 1962. The motility of the pelvic colon. II. Paradoxical motility in constipation and diarrhoea. Gut 3: 342–348.

17. Wangel AG, Deller DJ. 1965. Intestinal motility in man. III. Mechanisms of constipation and diarrhoea with particular reference to the irritable colon syndrome. Gastroenterology 11: 577–590.
18. Chowdury AR, Dinoso VP, Lorber SH. 1976. Characterization of a hyperactive segment at the rectosigmoid junction. Gastroenterology 71: 584–588.
19. Meunier P. 1986. Physiologic study of the terminal digestive tract in chronic painful constipation. Gut 27: 1018–1024.
20. Martelli M, Devroede G, Arhan P, Duguay C. 1978. Mechanisms of idiopathic constipation: outlet obstruction. Gastroenterology 75: 623–631.
21. Preston DM, Lennard-Jones JE. 1985. Pelvic motility and response to intraluminal bisacodyl in slow-transit constipation. Dig Dis Sci 30: 289–294.
22. Halls J. 1965. Bowel content shift during normal defaecation. Proc Roy Soc Med 58: 859–860.
23. Sarna SK. 1975. Gastrointestinal electrical activity: terminology. Gastroenterology 68: 1631–1635.
24. Christensen J, Anúras S, Hauser RL. 1974. Migrating spike bursts and electrical slow waves in the cat colon: effect of sectioning. Gastroenterology 66: 240–247.
25. Caprilli R, Onori L. 1971. Origin, transmission and ionic dependence of colonic electrical slow waves. Scand J Gastroenterol 7: 65–74.
26. Huizing JD, Stern HS, Chow E, Diamant NE, El-Sharkawy TY. 1985. Electrophysiological control of motility in the human colon. Gastroenterology 88: 500–511.
27. Gill RC, Cote KR, Bowes KL, Kingma YJ. 1986. Human colonic smooth muscle: electrical and contractile activity in vitro. Gut 27: 293–299.
28. Taylor I, Darby C, Hammond P. 1978. Comparison of rectosigmoid myoelectrical activity in the irritable colon syndrome during relapses and remissions. Gut 19: 923–926.
29. Bueno L, Fioramonti J, Ruckebusch Y, Frezinos J, Coulom P. 1980. Evaluation of colonic myoelectrical activity in health and functional disorders. Gut 21: 480–485.
30. Sarna SK, Waterfall WR, Bardakjian BL, Lind JF. 1981. Types of human colonic electrical activities recorded postoperatively. Gastroenterology 81: 61–70.
31. Aaroson MJ, Freed MM, Burakoff R. 1984. Colonic myoelectrical activity in persons with spinal cord injury. Dig Dis Sci 30 295–300.
32. Krishnamurthy S, Schuffler MD, Rohrmann CA, Pope CE. 1985. Severe idiopathic constipation is associated with a distinctive abnormality of the colonic myenteric plexus. Gastroenterology 88: 26–34.
33. Almy TP, Tulin M. 1947. Alterations in colonic function in man under stress. I. Experimental production of changes simulating the 'irritable colon'. Gastroenterology 8: 616–626.
34. Almy TP, Hinkle LE, Berle BB, Kern F. 1949. Alterations in colonic function in man under stress. III. Experimental production of sigmoid spasm in patients with spastic constipation. Gastroenterology 12: 437–449.
35. Narducci F, Shape WJ, Battle WM, London RL, Cohen S. 1985. Increased colonic motility during exposure to a stressful situation. Dig Dis Sci 30: 40–44.
36. Sullivan M, Cohen S, Snape WJ. 1978. Colonic myoelectric activity in irritable bowel syndrome. New Engl J Med 298: 878–883.
37. Latimer P, Sarna S, Campbell D, Latimer M, Waterfall W, Daniel EE. 1981. Colonic motor and myoelectric activity: a comparative study of normal subjects, psychoneurotic patients and patients with irritable bowel syndrome. Gastroenterology 80: 893–901.

2. Constipation

2.1 Assessment and classification

W.R. SCHOUTEN, TH.J.M.V. VAN VROONHOVEN,
A.G.M. HOOFWIJK & D.L. WESTBROEK†

Introduction

Constipation is an age-old and worldwide problem. In ancient times the Chinese technique for handling the problem of constipation consisted of massaging the abdomen with wooden rollers (Figure 1).

Constipation is just a symptom, with different meanings to different patients. Some patients have infrequent bowel actions while others present themselves with difficult defaecation. In Western society normal subjects have a stool frequency varying from three bowel actions weekly to three bowel actions daily [1]. In a recent survey up to five per cent of an American population sample said that they pass two or fewer stools a week [2]. Therefore it seems reasonable to use the stool frequency as a clinical guide and to define constipation as 'an infrequent defaecation with fewer than two bowel actions weekly'.

In recent years new techniques for the investigation of colonic motility and defaecation mechanism have been developed. Based on the results of these studies it has been suggested that there might be an indication for a surgical approach to the distressing problem of constipation. Because this approach is still controversial, it seems to be appropriate to review the suggested indications for the use of surgery in the treatment of constipation and to discuss the results as reported in literature so far.

History

At the beginning of this century Sir William Arbuthnot Lane was probably the first to perform intestinal bypass or colectomy with ileo-rectal anastomosis in patients with 'chronic intestinal stasis' [3]. Lane attracted ridicule with his surgical approach and for many years his idea remained controversial. At the same time Sir Arthur Hurst demonstrated that failure of normal defaecation

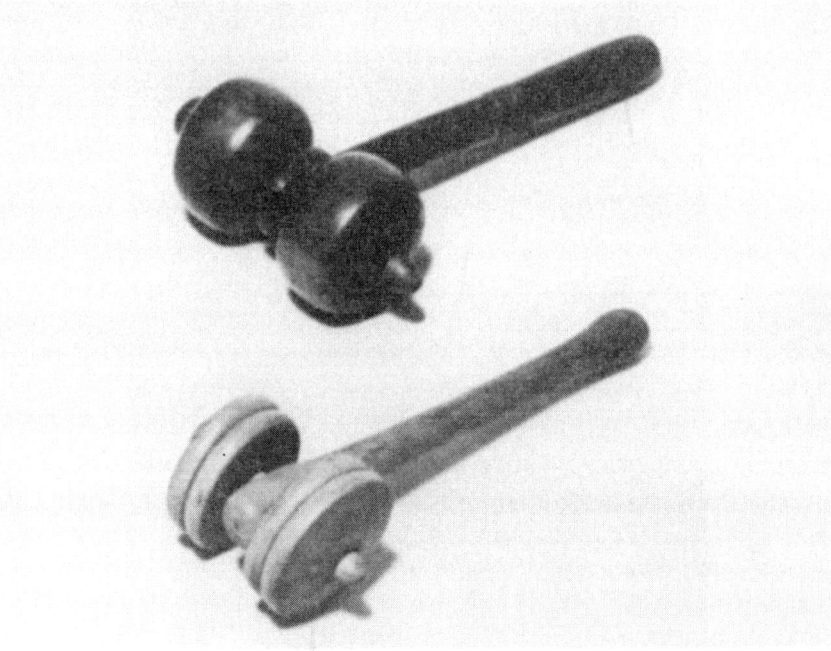

Figure 1. Wooden rollers for massaging the abdomen. The Chinese technique for handling constipation.

could be the cause of constipation. He proposed the term 'dyschezia' for this type of constipation due to an 'inability to defaecate completely'. He suggested that spasm of the anal sphincter muscles was responsible [4].

In the forties an attempt was made to treat patients with severe constipation, especially those with idiopathic megacolon, by performing bilateral lumbar sympathectomy. The rationale for this procedure was the presumption that constipation could be the result of autonomic nerve dysfunction. The results as reported in literature were very disappointing [5]. For many years idiopathic megacolon was regarded as the one and only indication for colectomy.

Up to a few years ago most surgeons were reluctant to remove a normal sized colon. Recently, three retrospective studies showed promising results after subtotal colectomy with ileo-rectal anastomosis in patients complaining of severe constipation with an apparently normal colon [6–8]. During the last two decades many authors suggested that constipation might be the result of ano-rectal outlet obstruction. This was based on the recognition that in some patients the internal sphincter muscle does not relax due to short segment aganglionosis, while in other patients the pelvic floor muscles do not relax during straining. In 1966 Bently reported the results of ano-rectal myectomy in patients with short segment Hirschsprung's disease with apparently good results [9].

At the same time Wasserman, and later on Wallace and Madden, proposed ano-rectal spasm (puborectalis syndrome) as a cause for constipation and reported their promising results of partial division of the puborectalis muscle [10, 11].

Investigation

Patient's history

An adequate history is mandatory in determining the patient's stool frequency. When a patient has fewer than two bowel actions a week the diagnosis of constipation may be considered. It is also necessary to determine the onset of symptoms because onset in childhood may suggest a congenital cause such as aganglionosis. Questions regarding dietary and bowel habits, the use of laxatives and prior abdominal or pelvic surgery may lead to the correct diagnosis. Characteristic symptoms such as prolonged and repeated straining at stool, rectal fullness, the sense of incomplete evacuation, the necessity of manual assistance and the loss of blood and mucus from the rectum may suggest a defaecation disorder.

Physical examination

Although in most patients with constipation physical examination will not reveal any pathological sign, a careful inspection of the ano-rectum is always mandatory to exclude ano-rectal pathology such as fissures, haemorrhoids, fistulous abscesses, rectocele and rectal neoplasm.

Endoscopic examination

In the vast majority of patients complaining of constipation endoscopic examination will not reveal any abnormality. However, some patients will demonstrate melanosis coli, while in other subjects a solitary rectal ulcer, sometimes associated with anterior mucosal prolapse, will be found. In constipation of recent onset endoscopic examination is indicated to rule out the presence of a neoplasm.

Biopsy

A rectal biopsy is indicated to confirm findings such as solitary rectal ulcer and aganglionosis. Although the value of the histopathological diagnosis of aganglionosis is well defined, there are still problems in the interpretation of biopsy material in the diagnosis of constipation of local neurogenic origin such as hypoganglionosis and short segment aganglionosis.

Barium enema

Especially in constipation of recent onset a barium enema is indicated to demonstrate or exclude organic abnormalities in the colon. In some patients with constipation barium enema films will reveal a redundant colon, while in other patients the width of the colon rather than its length is greater than normal. In a recent study the normal range for the width of the rectum and the colon has been established [12].

Defaecography

In the sixties cineradiography was developed for the dynamic investigation of defaecation mechanism. Some of the techniques used in that period were relatively complex, requiring time and sophisticated radiological equipment. At present simplified techniques such as defaecography and balloon proctogram are available. In several studies it has been shown that those techniques are reliable and simple to perform [13, 14]. It has been suggested that defaecography is more sensitive than clinical evaluation in the detection of defaecation disorders, associated with changes in the configuration of the rectum during straining such as anterior rectal wall prolapse, rectal intussusception and rectocele formation.

Colonic transit time study

A major step in the evaluation of constipation is the measurement of colonic transit time. Originally radiopaque markers were given on the first day. On day four and six, plain abdominal films were taken and the total number of markers were counted on each film [15]. At present most authors take daily films in order to establish the transit time of each segment of the colon. Normally all the markers have passed within seven days [16]. The transit time is prolonged when more than 20% of the markers are still present within the colon five days after ingestion. It is important to differentiate patients with a prolonged transit time from those with a normal transit time, because constipated patients with a normal transit of markers through the colon are mainly complaining of a defaecation disorder.

Ano-rectal manometry

It is generally supposed that ano-rectal manometry can be used as a simple and

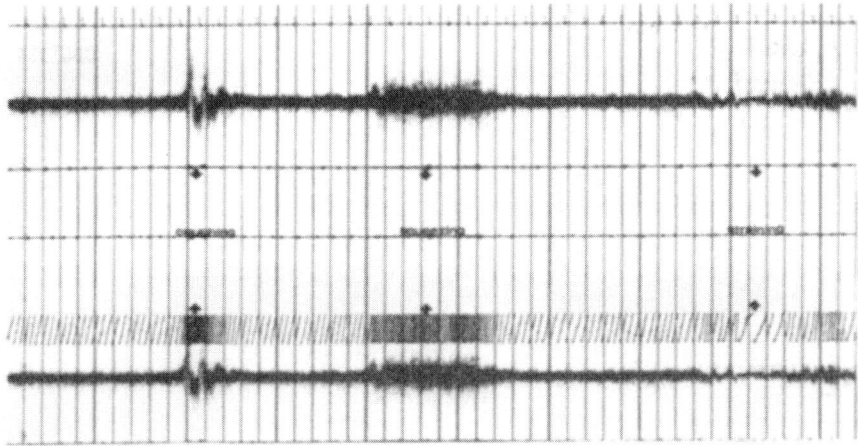

Figure 2. Normal activity of the puborectalis muscle at rest and during coughing, squeezing and straining.

reliable screening test in the diagnosis of Hirschsprung's disease, because in patients with aganglionosis the internal sphincter muscle does not relax upon rectal distension. In patients with non-Hirschprung constipation, however, ano-rectal manometry seems to be of little clinical value. Some authors have found manometric abnormalities in patients with idiopathic constipation, such as elevated resting pressure, reduced rectal compliance and reduced internal sphincter relaxation [17], while in other studies most manometric recordings were normal.

Electromyography

Electromyography is a reliable method for the investigation of the external anal sphincter and puborectalis muscles [18]. Normally at rest, a basal, low frequency activity will be recorded. During squeezing and coughing the muscular activity will increase, whereas during straining the activity of the puborectalis muscle decreases (Figure 2). In patients with a spastic pelvic floor syndrome a paradoxal increase in activity of the puborectalis muscle will be seen during straining (Figure 3).

Classification

Severe, chronic constipation may result from either colonic or ano-rectal outlet obstruction. Patients with colonic inertia have an apparently normal sized colon, while their whole gut transit time is markedly prolonged. In patients with ano-rectal outlet obstruction a normal colonic transit time will be

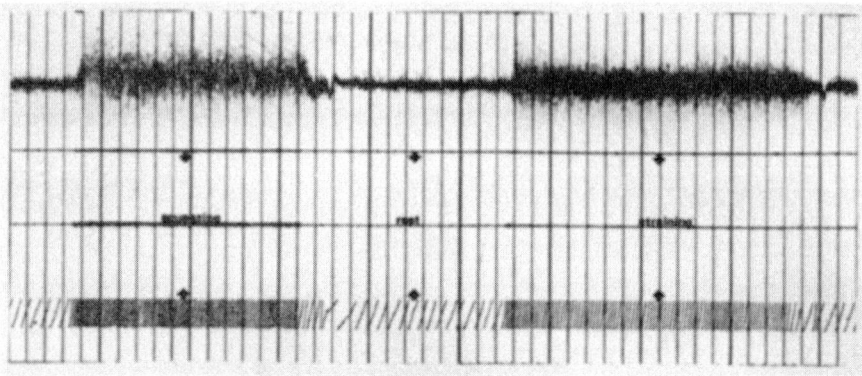

Figure 3. EMG-recording of the puborectalis muscle in a patient with spastic pelvic floor syndrome. Note the paradoxical increase of muscular activity during straining.

found; however, the radiopaque markers will accumulate in the rectum, indicating an evacuation difficulty. In order to select patients for surgical treatment a classification is necessary. Numerous classifications have been described and most attempts are either oversimplified or too detailed. The classification presented in Table 1 is also very comprehensive, and in our view quite useful for practical purposes.

Table 1. Classification of severe, chronic constipation.

I Slow transit constipation

II Ano-rectal outlet obstruction
1. Spastic pelvic floor syndrome:
   – alone
   – in association with:
   Solitary rectal ulcer
   Rectal intussusception
   Anterior mucosal prolapse
2. Short segment Hirschsprung's disease
3. Idiopathic megarectum or megacolon
4. Rectocele
5. Rectal intussusception
6. Painful anal stenosis (fissure, haemorrhoids, etc.)

References

1. Connell AM, Hilton C, Irvine C, Lennard-Jones JE, Misiewicz JJ. 1965. Variation of bowel habit in two population samples. Brit Med J 2: 1095–1099.
2. Drossman DA, Sandler RS, McKee DC, Lovitz AJ. 1982. Bowel patterns among subjects not seeking health care. Gastroenterology 83: 529–534.
3. Lane WA. 1908. The results of the operative treatment of chronic constipation. Br Med J I: 126–130.
4. Hurst A. 1909. Constipation and Allied Intestinal Disorders. Oxford University Press: 114–117.
5. Dixon CF, Judd DB. 1948. The surgical treatment of congenital megacolon. Surg Clin North Am: 889–901.
6. Hughes ESR, McDermott FT, Johnson WR, Polglase AL. 1981. Surgery for constipation. Aust NZ J Surg 51: 144–148.
7. Preston DM, Hawley PR, Lennard-Jones JE, Todd JP. 1984. Results of colectomy for severe idiopathic constipation in women (Arbuthnot Lane's disease). Br J Surg 71: 547–552.
8. Keighley MRB, Shouler P. 1984. Outlet syndrome: is there a surgical option? J Roy Soc Med 77: 559–563.
9. Bentley JRF. 1966. Posterior excisional ano-rectal myotomy in management of chronic faecal accumulation. Arch Dis Childhood 41: 144–147.
10. Wasserman JF. 1964. Puborectalis syndrome: rectal stenosis due to ano-rectal spasm. Dis Colon Rectum 7: 87–98.
11. Wallace WC, Madden WM. 1969. Experience with partial resection of the puborectalis muscle. Dis Colon Rectum 12: 196–200.
12. Preston DM, Lennard-Jones JE, Thomas BM. 1983. Towards a radiological definition of idiopathic megacolon. Gut 24: A488.
13. Mahieu P, Pringot J, Bodart P. 1984. Defaecography: I. Description of a new procedure and results in normal patients. Gastrointest Radiol 9: 247–251.
14. Mahieu P, Pringot J, Bodart P. 1984. Defaecography: II. Contribution to the diagnosis of defaecation disorders. Gastrointest Radiol 9: 253–261.
15. Hinton JM, Lennard-Jones JE, Young AC. 1969. A new method for studying gut transit times using radio-paque markers. Gut 10: 842–847.
16. Martelli H, Devroede G, Arhan P, Duguay C, Dormic C, Faverdin C. 1978. Some parameters of large bowel motility in normal man. Gastroenterology 75: 612–618.
17. Meunier P, Louis D, Jaubert de Beaujeu M. 1984. Physiologic investigation of primary chronic constipation in children: comparison with the barium enema study. Gastroenterology 87: 1351–1357.
18. Swash M, Snooks SJ. 1985. Electromyography in pelvic floor disorders. In: Henry MM, Swash M (eds) Coloproctology and the pelvic floor. London: Butterworths: 88–103.

2.2 Psychogenic causes in children

G. COREMANS & G. VANTRAPPEN

Introduction

Psychogenic constipation is a type of chronic constipation in children that is frequently associated with faecal soiling. It is considered as a specific entity by most authors [1–4]. The term 'psychogenic' may be inappropriate, as the pathogenesis of this type of faecal retention is most likely multifactorial [5–7]. Both physiological and psychological factors have a role in the pathogenesis. The psychological need for conservation of the symptom is not always clearly present and emotional problems may be the consequence as well as the cause of the chronic constipation and soiling. This condition has also been called functional megacolon, non-Hirschsprung's or pseudo-Hirschsprung's mega-rectum, chronic idiopathic constipation and colonic inertia. Other names are anal achalasia, congenital constipation and retentive encopresis. Tobon and Schuster introduced the term idiopathic megacolon since it does not refer to an aetiology when the cause is still unknown [4]. Psychogenic constipation is frequently accompanied by repeated involuntary passage of stool in the clothes, without there being any organic cause. This embarrassing symptom had been referred to as encopresis, faecal soiling or functional incontinence. Much of the confusion in the literature on these terms rests on the fact that they are used in cases with and without constipation [8, 9].

Incidence

Disorders of defaecation account for about 3% to 20% of the medical referrals in paediatric practice [10, 11]. Among children with a primary complaint of constipation Mercer found that about 65% had psychogenic constipation [12]. In 7-year-old schoolchildren Bellman reported an incidence of encopresis of 1.5% [8]. In most series the boys outnumber the girls by 1.6 to 3.1 [8, 12–14]. However, Coekin and Gairdner in a group of children with constipation as the primary condition and secondary faecal soiling, found an equal sex incidence [15].

Clinical manifestations

Psychogenic constipation usually has its onset about the time that toilet training begins. By the time the child is brought to the doctor, bowel movements occur at intervals of three to five days with occasionally a delay of up to three weeks. The outsize stools are passed with great difficulty and may cause plumbing problems by plugging the toilet. Many of these children display attempts to withhold bowel movements such as squeezing while in upright position [7]. Typically they keep their thighs rigidly adducted while having bowel movements in unusual and hidden places. Soiling between the evacuations is the dominant manifestation in 55% to 71% of the cases [10, 13, 14, 16]. Leakage occurs many times a day or even permanently. It usually ceases for a few days following a bowel movement and becomes progressively more severe as stool accumulates in the rectum. Soiling most of the time occurs during the day and worsens if the child exercises. The consistency of the leaking material is loose to claylike and has an unusual foul odour. The majority of the children are intelligent having good-to-average school performance. A significant number of them, however, have psychological problems and behaviour disorders [13]. The children are not infrequently socially withdrawn and submissive. Various neurotic signs are commonly seen in the parents, particularly in the mother [6, 17]. The mother is defined by Mercer as compulsive, meticulous, rigid and demanding in many ways [12]. This rigidity and compulsiveness are often manifested by coercive bowel training. The majority of children with idiopathic megarectum remain physically healthy. On examination a mildly distended abdomen is visible and faecal masses can readily be palpated. Not seldom soiling of the perineum is apparent. Faecal material protruding out of the anal opening is often seen on inspection. Rectal examination that is accomplished with unusual ease reveals the presence of semi-liquid to rocky hard faeces. Up to 80% of these youngsters have a colon full of faeces on plain roentgen film [16] (Figure 1). These children, when examined by barium enema show a widening of the rectum or even of the whole distal colon. The rectum is typically distended down to the anal canal (Figure 2).

Complications

Children with rectal impaction are seldom complaining of malaise, headache or impaired concentration, which are so frequently experienced by adults.

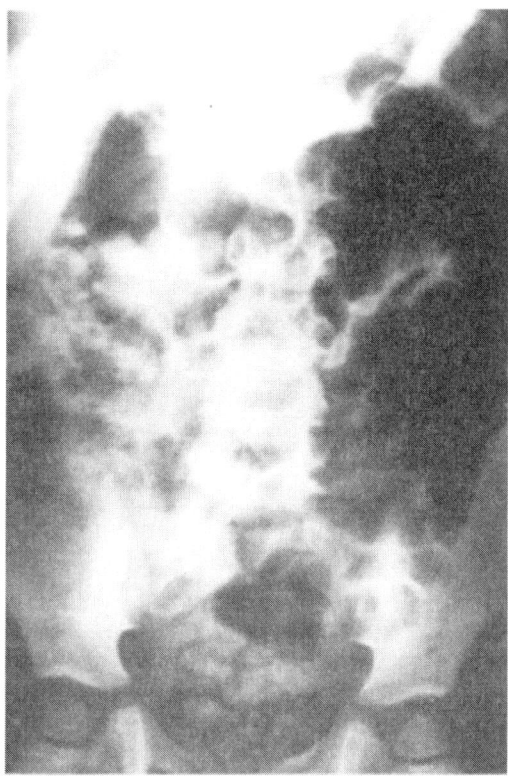

Figure 1. Plain roentgen film of the abdomen of a 4-year-old boy with constipation and faecal soiling. The distal colon is impacted with faeces. Accumulation of air proximal to the impaction is clearly visible.

However, reluctance to eat, failure to thrive, attacks of abdominal colics or vomiting and distension of the abdomen by gas may occur [14, 18]. Clinical pattern of acute intestinal obstruction has been reported [16]. The association of rectal impaction and uninhibited bladder contractions with enuresis has been described [19]. Obstructive uropathies are not uncommon in children with rectosigmoid impactions [5, 6, 20]. Recurrent urinary tract infections are common, particularly in girls with faecal soiling of the perineum [4, 5, 14, 21].

Diagnosis and differential diagnosis

As the psychological factors which are associated with disordered defaecation and faecal soiling in children with constipation of different cause, may obscure an underlying organic disease, careful investigation is important. Evaluation of the child begins with a thorough history and physical examination. A

74

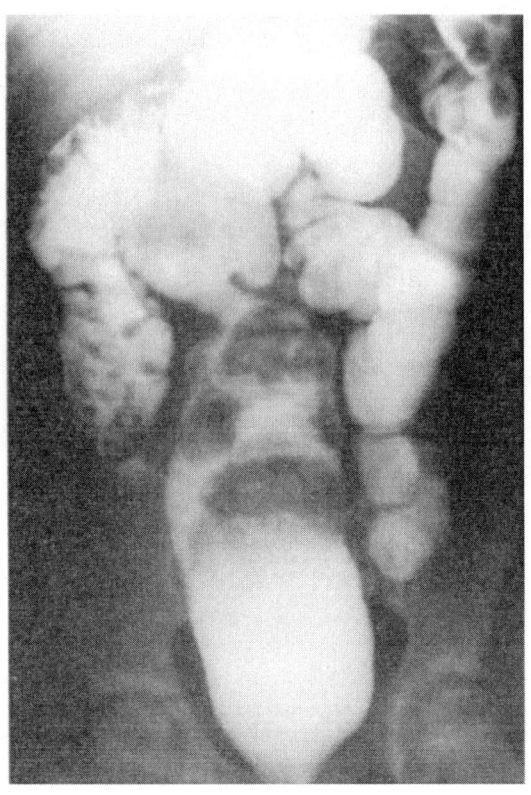

Figure 2. Barium enema in a 13-year-old boy with severe constipation and soiling, showing severe widening of the whole distal colon and distension of the rectum down to the anal canal.

developmental history and mental status examination including an estimate of the child's intelligence is recommended [1]. The parent observation that the child presents with a behaviour of grunting and flushing in the standing position in an attempt to hold stool is a crucial factor in the diagnosis of psychogenic constipation [1]. Careful history, physical examination and appropriate blood tests allow to rule out most other causes of chronic constipation which are summarized in Table 1.

Although neurologic abnormalities are uncommon in children with chronic constipation with or without soiling, manometry of the anorectum is very useful in excluding Hirschsprung's disease and spinal cord dysfunction. In the latter, clinical examination can already reveal associated skin pits or sinuses.

Manometric studies in constipated children reveal abnormalities in up to 10% of the patients [11, 22, 23]. Apart from classical Hirschsprung's disease, anal manometry can rule out other rare specific conditions such as 'ultra-short segment Hirschsprung's disease'. Failure of the internal anal sphincter to relax on rectal distension is a finding that should be interpreted cautiously in psychogenic constipation. Children with functional megarectum may show impaired sphincteric function because of the chronic distension of the rectal wall and one should be reluctant to make the diagnosis of 'ultra-short Hirschsprung's disease'.

A relapse of retentive soiling after adequate treatment calls for a biopsy with histochemistry and a barium enema, to make sure that organic disease has not been overlooked. A biopsy may provide the diagnosis of Hirschsprung's disease. The yield of a biopsy, however, is very low even in cases in which the symptoms have not regressed despite adequate treatment.

Roentgenograms in children with psychogenic constipation are normal, except for the large size of the colon and distension down to the anal canal. Barium enema is useful when signs of classical Hirschsprung's disease are present. The examination, however, should be done on an unprepared colon since enemas tend to obscure the transition between the colon and the narrow segment.

Urine analysis should be carried out routinely, particularly in girls. In cases with recurrent urinary infections or enuresis a roentgen examination of the urinary tract may be indicated.

Table 1. Classification of constipation in children.

Cause outside the colon	Cause in the ano-rectum and colon

– Lack of faecal bulk
  undernutrition
  lack of dietary fiber
– Chronic intake of medication
  Codeine, anticholinergics,
  antihistaminics, tricyclic anti-
  depressants, aluminium antacids
– Central nervous system disorders
  mental retardation, cerebral palsy, spinal
  cord anomalies (meningomyelocele,
  diastematomyelia)
– Impaired function of the muscles involved
  in defaecation
  amyotonia congenita, infectious
  polyneuritis, polyomyelitis, agenesis of
  abdominal musculature
– Metabolic dysfunction
  hypothyroidism
  thiamine deficiency
  porphyria
  infantile renal acidosis
  diabetes insipidus
  idiopathic hypercalcaemia
	– Acquired disease of the anus
	  chronic anal fissure or fistula
	  chronic perianal dermatitis
	  postsurgical stricture
	  Crohn's disease
	– Congenital disease
	  imperforate anus and associated recto-
	  perineal fistula
	  simple anterior displacement of the anus
	  anal or rectal stenosis
	  aganglionic megacolon
	  'ultra-short segment Hirschsprung's
	  disease'
	  presacral teratoma and rectal duplication
	  idiopathic slow colonic transit
	  impaired colonic propulsion
	  colonic neurofibromatosis
	  juvenile neural lipidosis with idiocy

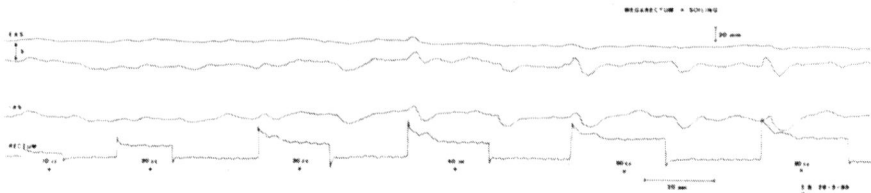

Figure 3. Increased rectosphincteric reflex threshold volume (40 cc) and decreased amplitude of the internal anal sphincter (IAS) relaxations in an 8-year-old boy with severe functional megarectum and continuous faecal soiling. The conscious rectal sensitivity threshold is normal (10 cc).

Pathogenesis

The pathogenesis of idiopathic megacolon is most likely multifactorial, involving multiple physiological and psychological factors. Furthermore, as in other chronic illnesses of childhood, the boundary between physical and emotional factors is often indistinct.

Manometric studies of the anorectum yield conflicting results and it is still not clear whether the abnormalities that have been found are the cause or the result of chronic faecal retention [10, 14, 16, 24–30].

Most authors found a normal or elevated anal resting tone [14, 16, 24, 28, 29]. In contrast, Loening-Baucke and Younoszai [10] and Reuter and Kaiser [30] found that the mean anal resting tone in children with constipation was lower than in control children. These conflicting results may be related to differences in recording techniques, differences in assessment of the recordings and to differences in patient populations. Arhan et al. observed that spontaneous variations of the resting pressure in the upper anal canal occurred more often in constipated patients than in control children [16]. Several investigators reported higher rectosphincteric reflex threshold volumes in children with functional megacolon [14, 16, 26, 31]. This finding implies higher volumes and higher pressures in the rectum are needed to produce relaxations of the internal anal sphincter (Figure 3). In contrast, Meunier et al. and Loening-Baucke and Younoszai found no significant difference between the mean rectosphincteric reflex threshold volume in constipated and control children [10, 24, 25] (Figure 4).

A decreased amplitude of the threshold inhibitory reflex also has been reported, indicating that the percentage of relaxation of the rectosphincteric reflex after rectal distension with a given volume is lower in constipated children than in control children [10, 14, 26]. Studies of Meunier et al. indicate that the conscious rectal sensitivity threshold in children with megarectum is increased, whereas the rectosphincteric reflex threshold volume is normal

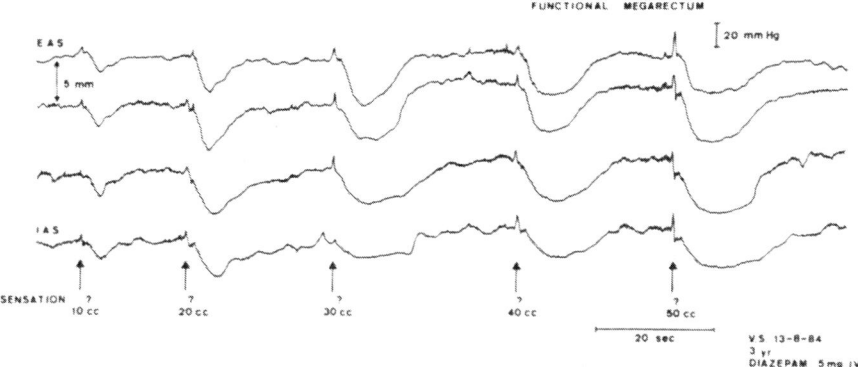

FUNCTIONAL MEGARECTUM

Figure 4. Normal relaxations of the internal anal sphincter (IAS) on repeated rectal distension in a 3-year-old boy with functional megarectum. The conscious rectal sensitivity threshold could not reliably be determined.

[24]. Such a situation clearly predisposes to soiling. Meunier et al. believe that, at the onset faecal retention occurs for psychological reasons to such a degree that impaction results. Distension of the rectum by the faecoloma lowers conscious rectal sensitivity and allows soiling as the rectosphincteric reflex threshold volume remains unaffected. The incidence of soiling increases proportionally to the decrease in conscious rectal sensitivity [24]. These important findings have been confirmed by Molnar et al. [11].

Callaghan and Nixon [26] and Porter [27] observed in children and adults with functional megarectum that a stage of enlargement may be reached at which distension causes relaxation of the external sphincter before any sensation is felt. This situation also clearly favours soiling.

The effect of adequate treatment on the ano-rectal variables in children with functional megarectum is still a matter of debate. Cucchiara et al. [14] noted a significant increase in amplitude of threshold inhibitory reflex and a reduction of rectal compliance after successful treatment. In contrast, Loening-Baucke found that the anal resting tone and the mean percentage relaxation of the rectosphincteric reflex remained significantly lower in both the recovered and not recovered constipated children with soiling. This finding led her to believe that the underlying cause of chronic constipation is the decreased ability of the internal anal sphincter to relax resulting in rectal distension. She further assumes that the low anal resting pressure may be responsible for the soiling [32].

It is not yet clear whether or not personality disorders are more frequent in these youngsters and their mothers than in controls. Identifiable psychological difficulties were reported in only 5% to 20% of these children and psychotherapy alone has yielded disappointing results [4, 8, 13, 33]. Levine's finding that children without constipation and soiling are exposed to similar stressful situations as children with psychogenic constipation, calls into question a suggested relationship between stressful life experiences and this disorder [34, 35].

At the present time it is not possible to determine whether emotional disturbances are the cause of stool retention or are secondary to the constipation and the soiling. Most authors believe that the emotional problems are an after-the-fact finding, simply because the child really does not know what to do about the bowel problems. Furthermore, the emotional disturbances seem to disappear with relief of the constipation [33, 36, 37].

Most likely both physiologic and psychological factors have a role in the pathogenesis of the disease. The relative importance of each of these factors is unknown. Fitzgerald proposed that painful defaecation is often the cause of a withholding pattern and that psychological factors may contribute to it [37]. They found no significant correlation between factors involved in toilet training and psychogenic constipation.

According to Bellman, psychogenic constipation seems to result from a complex interaction between factors such as relative developmental immaturities, coercive pot training, aggressive reactions of the parents on what may be normal soiling accidents, the emotional relationship between mother and child during the period when control of defaecation is learned and mental disease in one of the parents [8]. Also according to the hypothesis that psychogenic constipation with soiling is a multifactor disease Bemporad et al. identified a matrix of factors including certain developmental immaturities, early toilet training, a family characterized by personality disorders and a patient who develops a negativistic personality style with soiling utilised as a response to family conflicts [38].

Management

Because the aetiology of psychogenic constipation is still obscure, the various modes of therapy remain empirical and not always successful. The most effective treatment appears to be a combination of bowel cleansing with behaviour modification [3, 7]. The initial step consists of vigorously cleaning the colon impaction using hypertonic phosphate enemas followed by bisacodyl suppositories. Once the colon has been cleansed, mineral oil or lactulose in sufficient amounts to obtain liquid bowel movements, is prescribed. A possible hazard of mineral oil is that it may be carcinogenic and that it interferes with fat soluble vitamine absorption when given for long periods of time. Mineral oil pneumonia from aspiration in an unwilling child is a real danger. The initial dose is tapered off over a three to six month period. Meanwhile a fiber rich diet is encouraged and the child is required to visit the bathroom every day after breakfast, whether or not he feels the urge. A system of reward for bowel movements into the toilet is instituted. When this treatment modality fails, a number of alternatives including hospitalization, anal dilatation, anal myomectomy, biofeedback training and intensive psychotherapy have been proposed [22]. Schandling and Desjardins [33] obtained good results with myomectomy in nine of 11 children with severe constipation which was resistent to all non-surgical attempts of therapy. The rationale for the operation is to modify the forces tending to prevent evacuation. Olness et al. reported good to excellent results in 38 of 40 children with intractable constipation and soiling by giving biofeedback for the purpose of achieving anal sphincter control. Biofeedback training is not recommended as the initial treatment modality [39].

Routine referral of all constipated children with soiling to psychiatric or psychological therapy is to be avoided. Simple psychiatric counselling such as can be offered by the family physician will often suffice. Initial counselling by reassuring the children and the parents is very important. A positive, non accusatory approach should be pursued. Some authors believe that psychotherapy is more appropriately directed in the first place to the parents than to the child [40]. Silber advises an approach by which pressure on the child is reduced by a series of measures such as avoiding unnecessary discussions with the child about his bowel habits and incontinence [1].

The child with constipation and soiling who does not respond to physical therapy and who continues to resist to toileting may be an indication for evaluation by a paediatric psychiatrist. In case of serious family psychopathology or active parental opposition, psychiatric help may be necessary. Play therapy and conversion based on psychoanalytic methods often lead in these difficult cases to lasting results [8, 17]. It has to be stressed that psychotherapy cannot be a substitute for bowel cleansing, laxatives and a training program.

Outcome

In psychogenic constipation both the remission rate and the relapse rate are high. Management is difficult; not infrequently it takes a year to solve the problem of constipation with soiling in a child [41]. The presence of soiling seems to be a predictor of poor outcome [13]. Forty-seven to 100% of the children with psychogenic constipation can be successfully managed by medical treatment and toilet training [7, 13–15, 42, 43]. In all the major series reported in the literature poor patient compliance is blamed for less good results [8, 13, 14].

The reported relapse rate is as high as 15% to 20% and many children require treatment for three years or more [13]. Most authors found complete resolution of the symptoms by the onset of puberty [8, 13]. It is possible that symptoms would resolve with age in all these children regardless of treatment.

References

1. Silber DL. 1969. Encopresis. Discussion of aetiology and management. Clin Paediat 8: 225–231.
2. Bodian M, Stephens FD, Ward BCH. 1949. Hirschsprung's disease and idiopathic megacolon. Lancet i: 6–11.
3. Levine MD. 1981. The schoolchild with encopresis. Paediatrics in Review 2: 285–290.
4. Tobon F, Schuster MM. 1974. Megacolon: special diagnostic and therapeutic features. Hopkins Med J 135: 91–105.
5. Fitzgerald JF. 1977. Difficulties with defaecation and elimination in children. Clin Gastroenterol 6(2): 283–297.
6. Levine MD. 1982. Encopresis: its potentiation, evaluation and alleviation. Paediatr Clin North Am 29(2): 315–330.
7. Davidson M, Kluger MM, Bauer CH. 1963. Diagnosis and management in children with severe and protracted constipation and obstipation. J Paediatr 62: 261–275.
8. Bellman M. 1966. Studies on encopresis. Acta Paediat Scand (suppl.) 170: 1–138.
9. Berg I, Jones KV. 1964. Functional faecal incontinence in children. Arch Dis Child 39: 465–471.
10. Loening-Baucke VA, Younoszai MK. 1982. Abnormal anal sphincter response in chronically constipated children. J Paediatr 100(2): 213–218.
11. Molnar D, Taitz LS, Urwin OM, Wales JKH. 1983. Ano-rectal manometry results in defaecation disorders. Arch Dis Childh 58: 257–261.
12. Mercer RD. 1967. Constipation. Paediatr Clin North Am 14: 175–185.
13. Abrahamian FP, Lloyd-Still JD. 1984. Chronic constipation in childhood. A longitudinal study of 186 patients. J Paediatr Gastroent Nutrit 3: 460–467.
14. Cucchiara S, Coremans G, Staiano A, Corazziari E, Romanello G, DiLorenzo C, Tamburrini O, Auricchio S. 1984. Gastrointestinal transit time and anorectal manometry in children with fecal soiling. J Paediatr Gastroent Nutrit 3: 545–550.
15. Coekin M, Gairdner D. 1960. Faecal incontinence in children. Brit Med J 22: 1175–1180.
16. Arhan P, Devroede G, Jehannin B, Faverdin C, Révillon Y, Lefevre D, Pellerin D. 1983. Idiopathic disorders of faecal continence in children. Paediatrics 71(5): 774–779.
17. Pinkerton P. 1958. Psychogenic megacolon in children: the implications of bowel negativism. Arch Dis Child 33: 371–380.
18. Bently JFR. 1971. Constipation in infants and children. Progress Report. Gut 12: 85–90.
19. O'Regan S, Yazbeck S, Schick E. 1973. Constipation, bladder instability, urinary tract infections. Paediatrics 52: 241–245.
20. Shopfler CE. 1968. Urinary tract pathology associated with constipation. Radiology 90: 865–877.
21. Neumann PZ, de Domenico IJ, Nogrady MB. 1979. Constipation and urinary tract infections. Paediatrics 52: 241–243.
22. Clayden GS, Lawson JON. 1976. Investigation and management of longstanding chronic constipation in childhood. Arch Dis Child 51: 918–923.
23. Show A, Basher P, Blair K. 1980. Ano-rectal manometry for evaluating defaecation disorders. Va Med 107: 366–370.

24. Meunier P, Marechal JM, De Beaujeu MJ. 1979. Recto-anal pressures and rectal sensitivity studies in chronic childhood constipation. Gastroenterology 77: 330–336.

25. Meunier P, Pollard P, Marechal JM. 1976. Physiopathology of megarectum: the association of megarectum with encopresis. Gut 17: 224–227.

26. Callaghan RP, Nixon HH. 1964. Megarectum: physiological observations. Arch Dis Child 39: 153–157.

27. Porter NH. 1961. Megacolon: a physiological study. Proc R Soc Med 54: 1043–1047.

28. Holschneider AM, Mezler EM. 1974. Manometrische Studien zur anorektaler Kontinenz im Kindesalter. Brun's Beitr Klin Chir 221: 516–524.

29. Suzuki H, Armano S, Honzumi M et al. 1980. Recto-anal pressure and rectal compliance in constipated infants and children. Kinderchir 29: 330–336.

30. Reuter I, Kaiser G. 1976. Betrachtungen zum anorektalen Druckprofil. Helv Paediatr Acta 31: 141–148.

31. Schuster MM. 1973. Diagnostic value of anal sphincter pressure measurements. Hosp Prac 8: 115–119.

32. Loening-Baucke VA. 1984. Abnormal recto-anal function in children recovered from chronic constipation and encopresis. Gastroenterology 87: 1299–1304.

33. Schandling B, Desjardins JG. 1969. Anal myomectomy for constipation. J Paediatr Surg 4(1): 115–118.

34. Levine MD. 1975. Children with encopresis: a descriptive analysis. Paediatrics 56: 412–416.

35. Olatawura MO. 1973. Encopresis. Acta Paediatr Scand 62: 358–364.

36. Hussain SA. 1984. Childhood psychiatric disorders with physical manifestations. Indian J Paediatr 51: 205–216.

37. Fitzgerald JF. 1977. Difficulties with defaecation and elimination in children. Clin Gastroenterol 6(2): 283–297.

38. Bemporad J, Kresh R, Asnes R, Wilson A. 1978. Chronic neurotic encopresis as a paradigm of a multifactorial psychiatric disorder. J Nerv Ment Dis 166: 472–479.

39. Ollness K, McParland FA, Piper J. 1980. Biofeedback: a new modality in the management of children with faecal soiling. J Paediatr 96(3): 505–509.

40. Gardner D. 1965. Incontinence of urine or faeces. Brit Med J 2: 91–94.

41. Jolly H. 1976. A paediatrician's view on the management of encopresis. Proc R Soc Med 69: 21–22.

42. Levine MD, Bakow H. 1976. Children with encopresis: a study of treatment outcome. Paediatrics 58: 845–854.

43. Schmitt BD. 1984. Encopresis. Primary Care 11(3): 497–511.

2.3 The solitary rectal ulcer syndrome

J.H.C. KUIJPERS

Introduction

Solitary rectal ulcer (SRU) and colitis cystica profunda (CCP) are uncommon benign rectal conditions. The solitary rectal ulcer consists of one or several shallow, well-demarcated ulcers, which vary in size. Their base is covered with a greyish-white slough, and their shape is usually irregular with raised or polypoid edges. The ulcers are surrounded by a hyperaemic and nodular mucosa. The name 'solitary ulcer' is misleading since there may be more than one ulcer, and there is a stage of the disease when no ulceration is present [1, 2].

Colitis cystica profunda is characterised by one or several broad-based polyps or nodules, covered over by an intact mucosa, although ulceration may occur. The nodules are caused by mucin filled cysts located deep to the muscularis mucosae. CCP may develop after colonic ulceration from various factors, and occurs throughout the colon. The term 'colitis cystica profunda' is therefore a purely descriptive term. By far the most common association is with the solitary rectal ulcer. CCP of the rectum is likely the end response to, and develops from, a rectal ulcer [2–4].

Microscopy

Although their macroscopical appearances differ considerably, the lesions have similar microscopical features. The lamina propria is obliterated and replaced by fibroblasts and muscle fibres, the muscularis mucosae is markedly thickened, and the epithelium shows considerable reactive hyperplasia. There may be erosion of the superficial mucosa. Epithelial elements may be displaced in the submucosa, and are prone to undergo cystic dilatations due to retention of mucus, which may be confused with infiltrating adenocarcinoma [1, 2].

84

Site

Both conditions occur between four and 15 cm from the anal verge. Foremost they are located within a few centimetres from the anal verge on the anterior rectal wall. This is the area of the rectum which is located directly above the upper end of the anal canal. The lateral and posterior rectal wall are less involved, and circular involvement is rare.

Symptomatology

Disorders of bowel habit are common among patients with SRU and CCP. Patients with SRU complain of an urge to defaecate, a feeling of incomplete evacuation, constipation, the need of excessive straining, and passage of blood and mucus. They may have perineal, ano-rectal, back or left iliac pain. Several patients perform self-digitation. Rectal prolapse and an insufficient sphincter function may be present. Patients with CCP have the same pattern of complaints. They also have discharge, urgency, tenesmus and perineal and abdominal pain. Rectal prolapse is present in several patients.

The solitary rectal ulcer syndrome

It is obvious that both lesions have the same microscopical characteristics, and present themselves with comparable symptoms and signs. They are therefore considered to be different manifestations of the same phenomenon, for which a confusing variety of synonyms (solitary ulcer, solitary ulcer syndrome, benign solitary rectal ulcer, colitis cystica profunda, proctitis cystica profunda, hamartomatous inverted polyp of the rectum, enterogenous cyst) exists. Therefore the name 'solitary rectal ulcer syndrome' (SRUS) has been proposed to describe this condition [3, 5]. Predomination of either cystic dilatation or ulceration determines the macroscopical appearance.

Aetiology

The cause of SRUS is unknown. Hamartomatous malformations, self-induced trauma, local infection and ischemia have been put forward as possible causes of SRUS, but the exact aetiology remains unclear. There are only a few proven facts about the aetiology.

85

Complete rectal prolapse

Complete rectal prolapse has been found to be associated with SRUS.
Madigan and Morson [1] reported association with complete rectal prolapse in
16%, Martin et al. [5] found a full-thickness circumferential rectal prolapse
beyond the anal verge in 34%, a prolapse to the level of the anal margin in
25%, and occult rectal prolapse in 14%. In the series described by Ford et al.
[6] circumferential rectal prolapse was found in 34% of patients. Keighley and
Shouler [7] reported the occurrence of rectal prolapse in patients with SRUS in
24%, Snooks et al. [8] in 35% and Stuart [3] in 54%.

It has been suggested that prolapse is the cause of SRUS, since the mucosal
lesions are situated on the anterior prolapsing rectal wall, and healing of
ulceration followed surgical correction.

Anterior rectal wall prolapse

Anterior rectal wall prolapse, not protruding beyond the anal verge, has also
been reported in patients with SRUS. Martin et al. [5] found anterior rectal
bulging in 11%, Ford et al. [6] reported a prolapse involving the anterior rectal
wall in 52%, and in the series reported by Keighley and Shouler [7], anterior
mucosal prolapse occurred in 33%. Anterior rectal wall prolapse, not protruding beyond the anal verge, is the most important feature of internal intussusception of the rectum. Internal intussusception is the early stage of complete rectal prolapse. The only anatomical difference between internal intussusception and complete rectal prolapse is that in the latter disorder, the intussusception has proceeded through the anal canal [9]. Its symptoms are mucous
discharge, a feeling of urge or 'something coming down', and a sensation of
incomplete evacuation. The feeling of urge is not caused by faeces, but by the
intussusception, that fills the lower rectum. It is therefore false. This fake
sensation puts them up to straining, which, apart from some accidental discharge of mucus, will be in vain, and will only result in an increase of urge
which, again, leads to more excessive straining.

There is a relation with SRUS. Ihre and Seligson found anterior rectal wall
abnormalities similar to SRUS in 50% of patients with internal intussusception
[9].

Internal intussusception is difficult to diagnose, since external prolapse does
not occur during straining. And even in experienced hands, the anterior wall
prolapse is palpable during rectal examination with the patient straining in
only 30% [9]. It can easily be diagnosed by defaecography. Since internal
intussusception is the precursor of complete rectal prolapse, both have the
same radiological features. During defaecation straining the intussusception
begins as an anterior rectal wall prolapse, a few centimetres above the anal

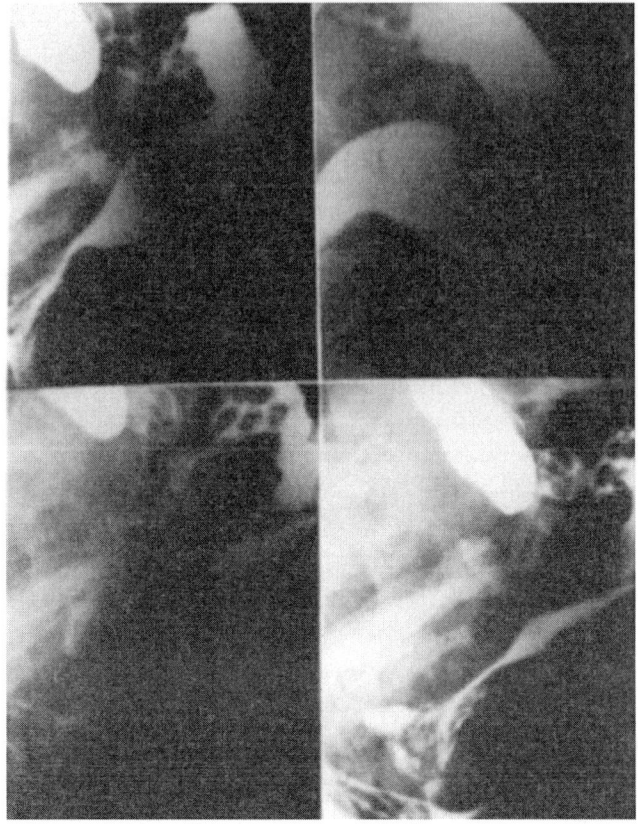

Figure 1. Internal intussusception. At rest the ano-rectal angle is normal, 90° (upper right). During straining the ano-rectal angle increases to about 150° (upper left). A prolapse of both the anterior and posterior rectal wall, not protruding beyond the anal canal, is seen (lower right). After straining has ceased, no more signs can be observed (lower left). (Reproduced with permission from Diseases of Colon and Rectum [14]).

canal, followed by a posterior wall prolapse at the same level. The prolapse finally becomes circular forming the intussusception. A typical funnel-like configuration can be seen (Figure 1) [10, 11]. The intussusception remains internal, in contrast to complete rectal prolapse, where it passes through the anal canal.

Pelvic floor dysfunction

Abnormal electromyographic behaviour of the pelvic floor musculature in patients with SRUS during straining has been reported by Rutter [12]. The normal response to straining consists of relaxation of the pelvic floor muscle, but in some patients with SRUS, he found that during defaecation straining

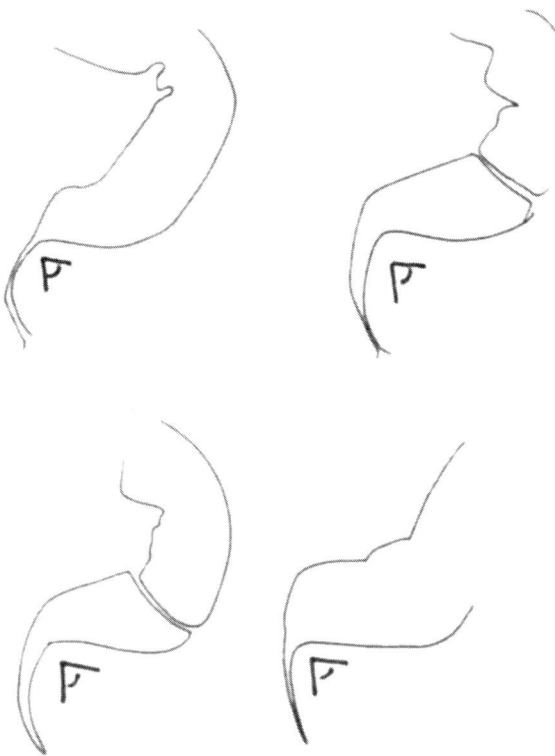

Figure 2. Spastic pelvic floor syndrome. At rest a normal ano-rectal angle of 90° is observed (upper right). During straining there is a slight descent of the ano-rectal level (upper left). The ano-rectal angle remains 90°, and does not increase (upper left, lower right). Barium is not excreted (lower left). (Reproduced with permission from Diseases of Colon and Rectum [14]).

the muscle went into a state of marked activity instead of relaxation, which persisted as long as the bearing down effort was maintained. This suggested that during straining the muscle contracted paradoxically, maintaining the ano-rectal angle. He found this abnormality in 77% of patients with SRUS, Lane [13] in 92%, Snooks et al. [8] in 50% and Kuijpers et al. [14] in 26%.

Kuijpers and Bleijenberg found this electromyographic abnormality in a group of patients who complained of severe constipation [15]. Defaecography in these patients revealed that the ano-rectal angle, which is a measure of pelvic floor function, remained 90° instead of increasing to about 135° (Figure 2). This confirmed a persistent contraction of the pelvic floor muscle during defaecation straining. Internal and external sphincter function was normal as demonstrated by anal manometry. They concluded that in these patients the anal canal was kept tightly closed during defaecation straining by a persistent contraction of a normal pelvic floor muscle (external sphincter). In another study [16] they demonstrated that 92% of patients with this pelvic floor dysfunction had segmental colonic transit abnormalities indicating outlet obstruction. They concluded, that this persistent contraction of the pelvic floor muscle represented a disorder of evacuation, a functional outlet obstruction. They proposed the name 'spastic pelvic floor syndrome'.

Patients with the spastic pelvic floor syndrome have difficulties with defaecation, or are unable to excrete faeces during several days, due to external sphincter contraction during straining. As a result, faeces accumulate in the rectum and more proximally in the colon, causing abdominal cramps and an increasing urge to defaecate. This increasing urge and the inability to defaecate lead to severe straining. Abuse of laxatives is common. Most patients can only empty their rectum by water enemas or by taking out the impacted faeces with their fingers.

Rectal digitation

Self-inflicted trauma has also been put forward as a possible cause of SRUS. In Madigan and Morson's series [1] 20% of patients admitted rectal digitation. Keighley and Shouler [7] mentioned that in their series 18% performed rectal digitation and suggested that they might have repeatedly traumatised their rectal wall during digital extraction of faecal material to assist defaecation. Ford et al. [6] reported that, 'on specific questioning', 48% of their patients admitted to inserting a finger into the anus to initiate defaecation. Thomson and Hill [17] found 'self-interference' in four out of six patients and concluded that, whether or not admitted, this was the most likely reason for ulceration.

It is much more likely, however, that it is performed because of a disorder of defaecation. It is done to initiate defaecation by opening the anal canal or to take out the presumed or impacted faeces.

Functional defaecation disorders

It has been stated that no clear pattern of bowel habit was emerged from patients with SRUS. Indeed, patients with SRUS present with a varied pattern of complaints, such as heavily straining, constipation, difficult and painful defaecation, a feeling of incomplete evacuation, and/or rectal digitation. Most patients have difficulties with defaecation for many years and admit a long past history of straining at stool.

More understanding of functional disorders of defaecation makes it likely, that these complaints are caused by either internal intussusception or the spastic pelvic floor syndrome. Since both disorders lead to straining, SRUS might well be the result of straining. In other words, the presence of SRUS indicates that these patients strain at stool. Straining in patients with either one of these disorders forces the mucosa of the anterior rectal wall into the anal canal, where it may repeatedly be damaged by anal sphincter pressure and rupture of overstretched submucosal vessels [2].

Although digital trauma cannot be completely excluded as a factor contributing to ulceration, it is obvious that digitation is performed because of a disorder of defaecation rather than from a desire to self-inflict trauma.

SRUS is therefore a traumatic lesion of the rectal wall, which is caused by straining due to a functional disorder of defaecation.

Diagnosis

Routine blood tests, and radiographs, including barium enema, make no contribution to the diagnosis, which is made on sigmoideoscopy, and confirmed by rectal biopsy. Biopsy is always mandatory to exclude carcinoma.

Examination of the perineal area while the patient strains, preferably in the squatting position, demonstrates the presence of a complete rectal prolapse. In patients without an overt prolapse, digital examination of the rectum during straining might reveal anterior rectal wall prolapse, which suggests the presence of internal intussusception [9].

Evaluation of pelvic floor activity during straining may reveal paradoxical contraction. Ask the patient to strain and observe whether the perineum descends. Feel whether anal pressure increases or decreases during straining, and whether the levator muscle relaxes or contracts.

Defaecography

Defaecography is the visualisation of the act of defaecation. It provides an exact anatomical image of changes in the rectal wall and pelvic floor function during defaecation straining, and is therefore a suitable procedure to detect functional disorders of defaecation [10]. Since disorders of defaecation are common among patients with SRUS, defaecography is indicated. Kuijpers et al. performed defaecography in 19 patients with SRUS and found functional disorders in 18 [14]. In 12 patients the rectum prolapsed without passing through the anal canal. Internal intussusception of the rectum was diagnosed. In five other patients the ano-rectal angle did not increase during defaecation straining, but remained 90°, indicating a persistent contraction of the pelvic floor muscle, which was confirmed by electromyography. These patients had spastic pelvic floor syndrome. One last patient had isolated anterior rectal wall prolapse.

Electromyography

Electromyography of the pelvic floor muscle in patients with SRUS may reveal paradoxical contraction during straining [8, 12, 15]. To exclude voluntary contraction during the examination due to embarrassment of the patient, segmental colonic transit time studies may be done. It reveals abnormal segmental transit times indicating outlet obstruction in about 90% of patients [16].

Treatment

Sulfasalazine and topical steroids are of no significant benefit to these patients, since it is a traumatic lesion. When investigation has demonstrated complete rectal prolapse or intussusception, it should be treated. A variety of procedures has been advocated to treat the prolapsing rectum, but posterior rectopexy appears to provide the best results. In most patients posterior rectopexy results in resolution of both symptoms and pathologic changes in the rectum [3, 5, 7, 14, 18]. When the prolapse has been treated and the SRUS persists, defaecography should be repeated to confirm adequate fixation to the sacrum. When a persistent intussusception had been excluded, EMG-studies should be performed to diagnose spastic pelvic floor syndrome. In the series reported by Kuijpers et al. 16% of the patients had both disorders [16]. Straining in patients with spastic pelvic floor syndrome may cause the rectum to loosen from the sacrum and to intussuscept, and after rectopexy the SRUS persists due to the outlet obstruction.

Treatment of the spastic pelvic floor syndrome is difficult. Subtotal colectomy in patients with delayed colonic transit time appears to be without benefit [15, 19]. Defaecation frequency increases, since colonic capacity is impaired, but the need to strain will persist, and the defaecation itself will remain difficult and painful. When colonic transit time is delayed in these patients, it must therefore be regarded as being caused by faecal retention due to outlet obstruction rather than by decreased colonic motility [16].

Good results of division of the puborectalis for a similar abnormality have been reported by several authors [20, 21], but the efficiency of this procedure in patients with the spastic pelvic floor syndrome is discussed [22]. The puborectalis sling is not that important in the retention of stools, since patients with a sphincter rupture have a normal puborectalis function and yet are incontinent. Contraction of this latter muscle fails to prevent unwanted evacuation. For this reason it is difficult to believe that the puborectalis muscle only is responsible for this defaecation disorder. Since the syndrome is caused by an abnormal function of a normal muscle, it should be possible for the patient to relearn how to relax the muscle during defaecation straining. This might be done by biofeedback.

Excellent results of biofeedback treatment have been found by Bleijenberg and Kuijpers in 10 patients (unpublished observation). It appeared to be a painless, but time-consuming procedure. All patients regained pelvic floor relaxation during defaecation straining. Eight patients were able to defaecate on a daily basis without straining or pain. However, two patients who had delayed colonic transit times in all segments, remained constipated. Subtotal colectomy in these two gave excellent results, which suggests that delayed colonic transit in all segments might be secondary to outlet obstruction.

Complications

Circular involvement and accompanying fibrosis may lead to radiological stenosis of the rectum, which is rarely symptomatic. The only life-threatening complication of SRUS is massive blood loss, which occurs in about 6% of patients [1, 5]. When intussusception is present, it probably will increase, and after a certain time it will protrude through the anus, resulting in complete rectal prolapse. The long periods of excessive and fruitless straining may lead to damage of the pudendal and perineal nerves. This will result in secondary neuropathic damage to the muscles and weakening of the pelvic floor muscle, resulting in either faecal incontinence or the descending perineum syndrome.

The descending perineum syndrome

It is a descriptive term for a group of patients with a distinct condition. When these patients strain at defaecation, their perineum balloons downwards and the pelvic floor occupies a lower position with reference to the bony plane than in normal controls [23]. This can be demonstrated by defaecography or by using an external device [24]. The syndrome is considered to be present, when the plane of the perineum descends beyond that of the ischial tuberosities during straining.

The most prominent and persistent feature is a pronounced difficulty with defaecation. They have a sense of obstruction and a feeling of incomplete evacuation, accompanied by a vague, dull, aching pain in the perineum and sacral region. Rectal digitation is frequently performed.

Some authors consider this feeling of obstruction to be caused by a prolapse of the anterior rectal wall, acting as a plug to block free passage of faeces through the anal canal [23], but EMG studies of the pelvic floor have revealed the same abnormal behaviour as in patients with the spastic pelvic floor syndrome [12, 16]. The external sphincter is innervated separately from the puborectalis muscle [25]. The nerves may be affected differently and occasionally even one group of nerves only may be affected. In patients with idiopathic faecal incontinence, histological and electrophysiological abnormalities have been demonstrated in the pelvic floor [26], but the external sphincter was affected more seriously than the puborectalis muscle. When the puborectalis muscle would be mainly affected, the perineum would descend lower than normal during straining, but continence would only slightly be impaired. In patients with the descending perineum syndrome anal pressures are indeed rather normal [27]. In these patients faecal continence is mainly dependent of external sphincter function, and it is obvious that haemorrhoidectomy and anal stretch procedures are contra-indicated since they may impair external sphincter function and result in faecal incontinence [27].

References

1. Madigan MR, Morson BC. 1969. Solitary ulcer of the rectum. Gut 10: 871-881.
2. Rutter KR, Riddell RH. 1975. The solitary rectal ulcer syndrome. Clin Gastroenterol 4: 505–530.
3. Stuart M. 1984. Proctitis cystica profunda. Incidence, aetiology and treatment. Dis Colon Rectum 27: 153–156.
4. Martin JK, Culp CE, Weiland LH. 1980. Colitis cystica profunda. Dis Colon Rectum 23: 488–491.
5. Martin CJ, Parks TG, Biggart JD. 1981. Solitary rectal ulcer syndrome in Northern Ireland, 1971–1980. Br J Surg 68: 744–747.
6. Ford MJ, Anderson JR, Gilmour HM, Holt S, Sircus W, Heading RC. 1983. Clinical spectrum of 'Solitary ulcer' of the rectum. Gastroenterology 84: 1533–1540.
7. Keighley MRB, Shouler P. 1984. Clinical and manometric features of the solitary rectal ulcer syndrome. Dis Colon Rectum 27: 507–512.
8. Snooks SJ, Nicholls RJ, Henry MM, Swash M. 1985. Electrophysiological and manometric assessment of the pelvic floor in the solitary rectal ulcer syndrome. Br J Surg 72: 131–133.
9. Ihre T, Seligson U. 1975. Intussusception of the rectum-internal procidentia: treatment and results in 90 patients. Dis Colon Rectum 18: 391–396.
10. Kuijpers JHC, Strijk SP. 1984. Diagnosis of disturbances of continence and defaecation. Dis Colon Rectum 27: 658–662.
11. Hoffman MJ, Kodner IJ, Fry RD. 1984. Internal intussusception of the rectum; diagnosis and surgical management. Dis Colon Rectum 27: 435–441.
12. Rutter KPR. 1974. Electromyographic changes in certain pelvic floor abnormalities. Proc R Soc Med 67: 53–56.
13. Lane RH. 1974. Clinical application of ano-rectal physiology. Proc R Soc Med 68: 28–30.
14. Kuijpers JHC, Schreve RH, Ten Cate Hoedemaker H. 1986. Diagnosis of functional disorders of defaecation causing the Solitary Rectal Ulcer Syndrome. Dis Colon Rectum 29: 126–129.
15. Kuijpers JHC, Bleijenberg G. 1985. The Spastic Pelvic Floor Syndrome, a cause of constipation. Dis Colon Rectum 28: 669–672.
16. Kuijpers JHC, Bleijenberg G, de Morree H. 1986. The Spastic Pelvic Floor Syndrome. Large bowel outlet obstruction caused by pelvic floor dysfunction: a radiological study. Int J Colorect Dis 1: 44–48.

17. Thomson H, Hill D. 1980. Solitary rectal ulcer: always a self-induced condition? Br J Surg 67: 784–785.
18. Schweiber M, Alexander-Williams J. 1977. Solitary-ulcer syndrome of the rectum. Its association with occult rectal prolapse. Lancet i: 170–171.
19. Preston DM, Hawley PR, Lennard-Jones JE, Todd IP. 1984. Results of colectomy for severe idiopathic constipation in women (Arbuthnot Lane's disease). Br J Surg 71: 547–552.
20. Wasserman I. 1964. Puborectalis syndrome (rectal stenosis due to ano-rectal spasm). Dis Colon Rectum 7: 87–98.
21. Wallace WC, Madden WM. 1969. Partial puborectalis resection: a new surgical technic for ano-rectal dysfunction. South Med J 62: 1123–1126.
22. Barnes PRH, Hawley PR, Preston DM, Lennard-Jones JE. 1985. Experience of posterior division of the puborectalis muscle in the management of chronic constipation. Br J Surg 72: 475–477.
23. Parks AG, Porter NH, Hardcastle J. 1966. The Syndrome of the Descending Perineum. Proc R Soc Med 59: 477–482.
24. Henry MM, Parks AG, Swash M. 1982. The pelvic floor musculature in the Descending Perineum Syndrome. Br J Surg 69: 470–472.
25. Percy JP, Swash M, Neil ME, Parks AG. 1981. Electrophysiological study of motor nerve supply of pelvic floor. Lancet i: 16–17.
26. Parks AG, Swash M, Urich H. 1977. Sphincter denervation in ano-rectal incontinence and rectal prolapse. Gut 18: 656-665.
27. Read NW, Bartolo DCC, Read MG, Hall J, Haynes WG, Johnson AG. 1983. Differences in ano-rectal manometry between patients with haemorrhoids and patients with Descending Perineum Syndrome: implications for management. Br J Surg 70: 656-659.

2.4 Surgical treatment

W.R. SCHOUTEN, TH.J.M.V. VAN VROONHOVEN,
A.G.M. HOOFWIJK & D.L. WESTBROEK†

Slow transit constipation

At the beginning of this century, Sir William Arbuthnot Lane was probably the first to perform colectomy with ileo-rectal anastomosis in patients with severe constipation [1]. For many years most surgeons were reluctant to remove an apparently normal colon and colectomy was only performed in patients with idiopathic megacolon (Table 1).

However, some studies show that patients with slow transit constipation showed no response to stimulation with a surface acting laxative. This finding suggests the possibility of a myenteric plexus disorder [7]. Examining resected colon specimens with a special silver staining technique, Preston et al. [8] demonstrated complete loss of the argyrophil plexus with a marked increase in Schwann cells indicating that extrinsic damage to the plexus had occurred. Based on these findings, these authors as well as others suggested that the myenteric plexus abnormality is not the primary cause, but may be the result of longstanding laxative use. Krishnamurthy et al. also found a distinctive abnormality of the myenteric plexus in twelve patients who underwent subtotal colectomy for constipation. Using conventional light microscopy (HE-staining) no abnormalities could be found. In contrast, silver stains (Smith's method) revealed distinctive changes in the myenteric plexus. These changes were different from those previously described in intestinal pseudo-obstruction [9].

These authors suggest that severe idiopathic constipation could be just another manifestation of chronic intestinal pseudo-obstruction and that these abnormalities may be developmental in origin [9].

In a retrospective study using the antineurofilament monoclonal antibody NF_2F_{11} we could demonstrate a disturbed extrinsic innervation in adult patients with severe constipation [10]. In normal bowel the axons of the myenteric and submucous plexus do stain with this monoclonal antibody (Table 2). Using this method in patients with Hirschsprung's disease, heavily stained axon bundles will be found [11]. Because in Hirschsprung's disease the intrinsic innervation is lacking, the stained axon bundles can only be of extrinsic origin. In patients with constipation and pseudo-obstruction a lack of axonal staining has been found. This indicates disturbed extrinsic innervation. In our view it is unlikely that this is a secondary phenomenon caused by laxatives, as the same picture was found in neonates with severe constipation, who have never been treated with laxatives [10]. Because slow transit constipation seems to be associated with a distinctive visceral neuropathy, partial or subtotal colectomy is probably a rational therapy for this type of constipation. However, the distribution of these neuropathologic changes along the gastro-intestinal tract in patients with slow-transit constipation and pseudo-obstruction has yet to be defined.

In three previous studies the results of subtotal colectomy in patients with severe constipation without megacolon are reported [1, 2, 3]. Although these results are apparently good (Table 1), the exact role of colectomy has yet to be defined.

Table 1. Results of colectomy in the treatment of constipation, as reported in literature.

Author	Treatment	Idiopathic constipation			
		with megacolon		without megacolon	
		n	Success (%)	n	Success (%)
Lane and	Subtotal colectomy	9	88		
Todd [4]	Hemicolectomy	2	50		
	Sigmoid resection	3	33		
McCready	Subtotal colectomy	6	100		
and Beart [5]	Hemicolectomy	5	100		
	Anterior resection	8	75		
Hughes et al. [1]	Subtotal colectomy	7	100	10	80
Belliveau et al. [6]	Subtotal colectomy	29	76		
Preston et al. [2]	Subtotal colectomy			16	87,5
Keighley and Shouler [3]	Subtotal colectomy			10	90

Editorial comment

The results of subtotal colectomy are unpredictable. In a few patients rectal evacuation remains impossible and some eventually require a stoma (4 out of 30 in my experience). There are a few patients who undergo colectomy for megacolon who subsequently develop a megarectum with recurrent constipation. Coeco-rectal anastomosis in these patients gives poor results because the coecum dilates. Five patients with gross megarectum have required an ileo-anal pouch anastomosis as the only means to prevent a permanent stoma with good results. Even if a megarectum does not develop, episodic diarrhoea or constipation is a problem in 20–30% of patients after subtotal colectomy and ileo-rectal anastomosis.

M.R.B. Keighley

Spastic pelvic floor syndrome; outlet obstruction

At the beginning of this century Sir Arthur Hurst demonstrated that failure of normal defaecation could be the cause of constipation [4]. For this type of constipation several terms have been proposed like 'dyschezia' and 'anismus'. Because Wasserman and Wallace et al. proposed spasm of the puborectalis muscle as a cause of constipation, they advocated partial division of puborectalis muscle for the treatment of this defaecation disorder [12, 13]. Although their early results were promising, two recent studies revealed very disappointing results after division of the puborectalis muscle (Table 3). Using defaecography or balloon proctography the characteristic findings of spastic pelvic floor syndrome have been recently defined [14–17]. In patients with impaired relaxation of the pelvic floor the ano-rectal angle does not increase during attempted straining, whereas the patient's failure to pass a balloon filled with barium suspension is another criterion for spastic pelvic floor

Table 2. Immunostaining with antineurofilament monoclonal antibody NF_2F_{11}.

		HE-staining	Antibody NF_2F_{11}
Normal colon	Ganglion cells	+	−
	Meissner axons	+	+
	Auerbach axons	+	++
Hirschsprung's disease	Ganglion cells	−	−
	Meissner axons	−	+++
	Auerbach axons	−	+++
Constipation	Ganglion cells	+	−
	Meissner axons	+	−
	Auerbach axons	+	−

syndrome. When recording activity of the puborectalis muscle a paradoxical increase in activity will be found in patients with this syndrome (see Figure 3; chapter 2.1). In our view spastic pelvic floor syndrome is the manifestation of a functional disorder of the pelvic floor muscles. Improvement will be rarely achieved by partial division of the puborectalis muscle. It has been suggested that biofeedback and relaxation training might be helpful in the treatment of these patients. We have so far treated five patients with spastic pelvic floor syndrome with relaxation training. Although this treatment is time consuming the preliminary results are very promising. Further investigation will be necessary to analyse if biofeedback and relaxation training can become a benificial treatment in patients with spastic pelvic floor syndrome.

Editorial comment

The results of ano-rectal myectomy for outlet obstruction have now been analysed in 34 patients. Spontaneous defaecation after operation was possible in 67% of patients and the use of laxatives was not required. These results were sustained in all patients having a satisfactory early response. The mechanism responsible for this improvement is not understood but the operation is associated with persistent fall in resting anal pressures. Apart from transient incontinence in one patient, there were no other complications. The operation seems therefore to be potentially beneficial in these patients.

M.R.B. Keighley

Rectal intussusception

Patients with ano-rectal outlet obstruction may have internal intussusception of the rectum. Whereas complete, external prolapse of the rectum can be demonstrated quite easily by clinical inspection, the diagnosis of internal intussusception is difficult to demonstrate either by physical examination or by endoscopic evaluation and barium contrast studies. It has been shown that

Table 3. Results of partial division of puborectalis muscle for spastic pelvic floor syndrome, as reported in literature.

Author	*n*	Success rate (%)
Wasserman (1964) [12]	3	100
Wallace and Madden (1965) [13]	44	100?
Keighley and Shouler (1984) [3]	7	14,3
Barnes et al. (1985) [15]	9	22,2

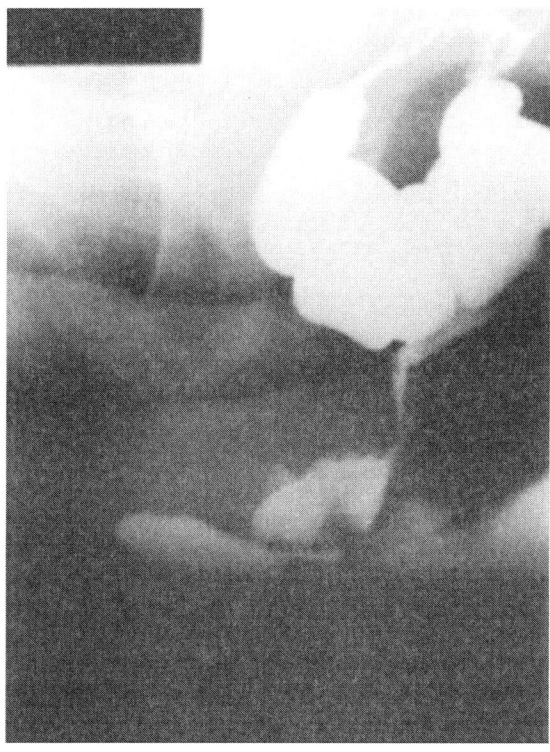

Figure 1. Defaecography in a patient with rectal intussusception (↓ distal part of the intussusception).

defaecography is the most useful diagnostic procedure to identify internal intussusception [18–21]. Evacuation proctography has revealed that the rectal wall begins to intussuscept into the lumen approximately 8 cm above the anal verge. A typical configuration will be seen (Figure 1). Because the intussusception does not pass beyond the anal verge it is called internal intussusception as opposed to complete prolapse of the rectum. It has been reported that internal rectal intussusception is much more common than complete rectal prolapse [22]. Women are affected six times more often than men, with a peak incidence for women in the fifth decade [23]. Patients with internal intussusception have difficult defaecation associated with tenesmus, rectal fullness, incomplete evacuation and occasional passage of blood and mucus per rectum. The intussusception might be associated with perineal descent, solitary rectal ulcer, spastic pelvic floor syndrome and rectocele. Because it has been suggested that internal intussusception is the precursor of complete rectal prolapse, its treatment should be identical. The results of surgical therapy, in patients with internal rectal intussusception, including rectopexy, sigmoid resection and Delorme's procedure, seems to be satisfying, as reported in literature (Table 4).

Table 4. Results of surgical treatment of rectal intussusception, as reported in literature.

Author	Therapy	*n*	Success rate (%)
Hoffmann et al. [19]	Rectopexy	8	100
Berman et al. [24]	Delorme	14	100
Kuijpers and de Morree [21]	Rectopexy	10	100

Editorial comment

The results of posterior rectopexy for incomplete intussusception in 12 patients have recently been reviewed. In all cases the radiological abnormality was adequately corrected by rectopexy but symptoms of tenesmus perineal pain and obstructed defaecation persisted in 8 of these patients. Although the early results are sometimes encouraging, relapse of symptoms is common and rectopexy, though logical is often associated with disappointing results.

M.R.B. Keighley

Hirschsprung's disease: ano-rectal myectomy

When classical Hirschsprung's disease is treated by restorative anterior resection of the rectum (Rehbein's procedure), a short aganglionic segment remains and symptoms of constipation will persist. It was found that these residual symptoms could be treated by ano-rectal dilatation. Based on these findings Bentley recommended ano-rectal myectomy for the treatment of short segment Hirschsprung's disease, which is one of the causes of ano-rectal outlet obstruction [24]. He assumed that the therapeutic effect of ano-rectal myectomy could be compared to the effect of gastro-esophageal myectomy (Heller's procedure) in patients with esophageal achalasia. Because his preliminary results were promising, other authors started to treat short segment Hirschsprung's disease by ano-rectal myectomy (Table 5).

Particularly in children and young adults the so-called 'idiopathic megarectum' may resemble short segment Hirschsprung's disease, clinically as well as radiologically. Therefore histological and manometric examination is necessary to differentiate between these two entities. In patients with idiopathic megarectum no abnormality of the intrinsic innervation will be found on routine histological examination and a normal internal sphincter reflex can be demonstrated. However, in several reports distinctive abnormalities of the intrinsic innervation such as hypoganglionosis and immaturity of the ganglion cells have been described, as well as histological abnormalities of the internal sphincter muscle [25–27]. It could be possible that 'idiopathic megarectum' is a

Table 5. 'Success rates' of ano-rectal myectomy as reported in literature.

Author	Short segment Hirschsprung		Non-Hirschsprung constipation	
	n	Success (%)	n	Success (%)
Bentley [25]	10	60	7	80
Thomas et al. [28]	11	40		
Nissen et al. [29]	11	91		
Lynn and van Heerden [30]	28	92		
Clayden and Lawson [31]	10	100	11	81,8
McCready and Beart [32]	13	61,5		
Shandling and Desjardins [33]			9	88
Martelli et al. [34]			62	77

transitional form towards short segment Hirschsprung's disease. Therefore it has been brought forward that ano-rectal myectomy might also be helpful in the treatment of patients with idiopathic megarectum.

The technique of ano-rectal myectomy consists of a submucosal resection of a 1 cm wide strip of internal sphincter muscle up to at least 6 cm above the dentate line. We have performed ano-rectal myectomy in 12 patients with severe constipation during the time period from 1982 to 1985. The patients ranged in age from 9 months to 23 years (mean age: 8.5 years).

Short segment Hirschsprung's disease was diagnosed in four patients and idiopathic megarectum was found in four patients. After a follow-up period varying from 3 to 35 months (mean follow-up: 25.1 months) the patients were reviewed and a success-rate of 75% was found (Table 6).

Table 6. Results of ano-rectal myectomy (St. Elisabeth Hospital, Tilburg).

Diagnosis	n	excellent (no. patients)	good (no. patients)	slightly improved (no. patients)
Hirschsprung after Rehbein's procedure	1	1		
Short segment Hirschsprung	4	1	3	
Idiopathic megarectum	4	3		1
Rest	3	1		2
Total	12	6	3	3

102

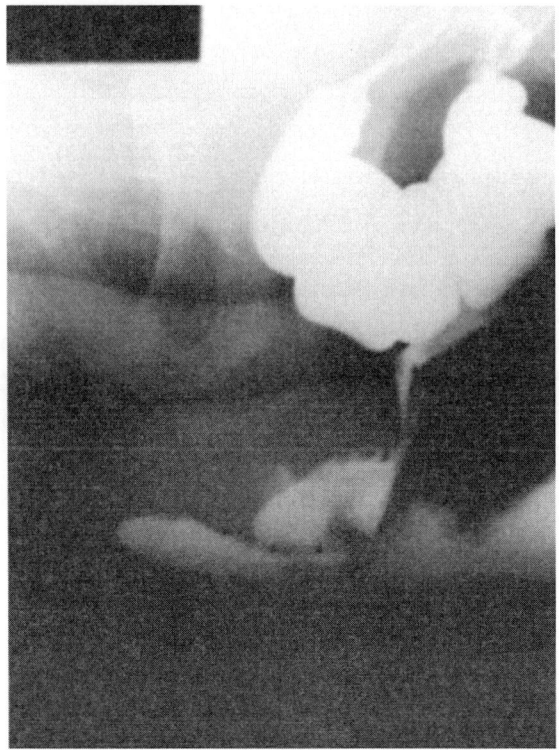

Figure 2. Defaecography in a patient with rectocele (↑).

Rectocele

Even in recent textbooks on coloproctology rectocele is not mentioned as a cause of defaecation disorders. Many surgeons do not realize that rectocele occurs frequently, especially in elderly multiparous women and is responsible for the distressing symptoms of ano-rectal outlet obstruction. Usually the rectocele does not become symptomatic until the fourth or fifth decade of life. The defect in the recto-vaginal septum, that may have existed for many years, becomes more prominent by progressive weakening of supportive tissues, as part of the aging process. During straining, the apex of the rectocele moves inferiorly and anteriorly. The stool will be entrapped in this sacculation and any further straining aggravates the problem by pushing the stool further from the anal opening. This mechanism can be demonstrated quite clearly on defaecography (Figure 2). Most patients with a symptomatic rectocele have a normal, daily urge to defaecate, but they 'can't get it out'. In order to empty their bowels some patients use manual pressure on the side or the front of the anal outlet or against the posterior vaginal wall. The rectocele may be associ-

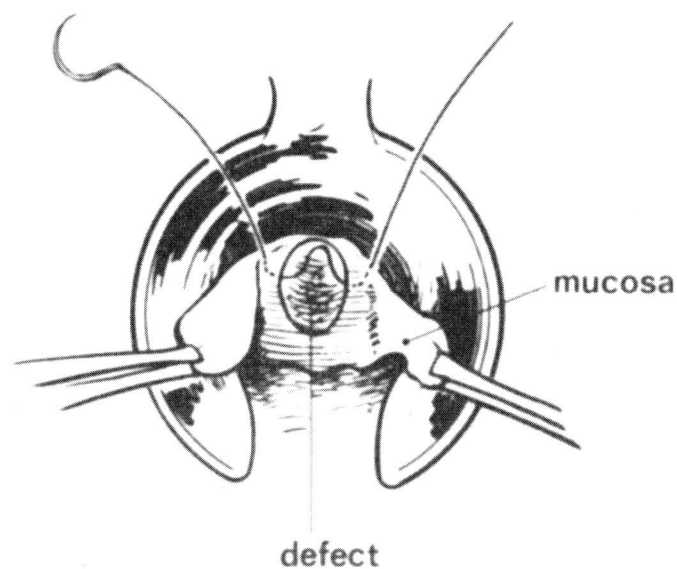

mucosa

defect

Figure 3. Schematic representation of trans-rectal repair of rectocele.

ated with other symptoms such as rectal fullness, incomplete evacuation, pain, bleeding, protrusion and soiling. The diagnosis is made by taking an adequate history and by bimanual recto-vaginal palpation. A hooked finger pressed on the anterior rectal wall can detect the pocketlike defect which is located just above the anal sphincter.

To confirm the diagnosis defaecography may be helpful (Figure 2). According to some authors transvaginal repair of the rectocele will not provide sufficient relief [35–38]. These authors recommend a combined recto-vaginal approach or a trans-rectal repair alone. For the trans-rectal repair the patient is placed in the prone jack-knife position. A midline incision is made starting at the dentate line and carried upward in the rectum approximately 7 to 8 cm. Mucosal flaps are developed on both sides. The musculo-fascial defect in the anterior rectal wall is closed with interrupted sutures (Figure 3). The mucosal flaps are then closed with a continuous suture. The results of this trans-rectal repair are promising (Table 7).

Table 7. Results of trans-rectal repair of rectocele as reported in literature.

Author	n	Follow-up (yrs)	Success rate (%)*
Sullivan et al. [38]	151	1.5	79.5
Capps [37]	51	?	94
Sehapayak [36]	355	?	84.5

* Success = excellent (asymptomatic) or good (considerable improvement).

104

Summary

In order to select patients with severe, chronic constipation for surgical treatment, evaluation and defining the different forms of constipation is necessary according to a standard protocol.

Surgical treatment seems to be beneficial especially for patients with slow transit constipation, short segment Hirschsprung's disease, idiopathic megarectum, rectocele and rectal intussusception. Further investigation will be necessary to define the exact role of the visceral neuropathy in the aetiology of slow transit constipation.

Finally it is possible that the so-called 'idiopathic' constipation does not exist at all.

References

1. Hughes ESR, McDermott FT, Johnson WR. Polglase AL. 1981. Surgery for constipation. Aust NZ J Surg 51: 144–148.
2. Preston DM, Hawley PR, Lennard-Jones JE, Todd JP. 1984. Results of colectomy for severe idiopathic constipation in women (Arbuthnot Lane's disease). Br J Surg 71: 547–552.
3. Keighley MRB, Shouler P. 1984. Outlet syndrome: is there a surgical option? J Roy Soc Med 77: 559–563.
4. Lane RHS, Todd JP. 1977. Idiopathic megacolon: a review of 42 cases. Br J Surg 64: 305–310.
5. McCready RA, Beart RW. 1980. Adult Hirschsprung's disease: results of surgical treatment at Mayo Clinic. Dis Colon Rectum 23: 401–407.
6. Belliveau P, Goldberg SM, Rothenberger DA, Nivatrongs S. 1982. Idiopathic acquired megacolon: the value of subtotal colectomy. Dis Colon Rectum 25: 118–121.
7. Preston DM, Lennard-Jones JE. 1985. Pelvic colon motility and response to intraluminal bisacodyl in slow transit constipation. Dig Dis Sci: 30: 289–294.
8. Preston DM, Butler MG, Smith B, Lennard-Jones JE. 1983. Neuropathology of slow transit constipation. Gut 24: A997.
9. Krishnamurthy S, Schuffler MD, Rohrmann CA, Pope CE. 1985. Severe idiopathic constipation is associated with a distinctive abnormality of the colonic myenteric plexus. Gastroenterology 88: 26–34.
10. Klück P, ten Kate FJW, Schouten WR, Bartels KCM, Tibboel D, van der Kamp AWM, Molenaar JC, van Blankenstein M. The efficacy of antibody NF_2F_{11} staining in the investigation of severe idiopathic constipation: Preliminary report. New Engl J Med: in press.
11. Klück P, van Muijen GNP, van der Kamp AWM, Tibboel D, van Hoorn WA, Warnaar SO, Molenaar JC. 1984. Hirschsprung's disease studied with monoclonal antineurofilament antibodies on tissue sections. Lancet 24i: 652–653.
12. Wasserman JF. 1964. Puborectalis syndrome: rectal stenosis due to ano-rectal spasm. Dis Colon Rectum 7: 87–98.
13. Wallace WC, Madden WM. 1969. Experience with partial resection of the puborectalis muscle. Dis Colon Rectum 12: 196–200.
14. Mahieu P, Pringot J, Bodart P. 1984. Defaecography: I. Description of a new procedure and results in normal patients. Gastrointest Radiol 9: 247–251.
15. Barnes PRH, Hawley PR, Preston DM, Lennard-Jones JE. 1985. Experience of posterior

division of the puborectalis muscle in the management of chronic constipation. Br J Surg 72: 475–477.

16. Kuijpers JHC, Bleijenberg G. 1985. Het spastische-bekkenbodem syndroom, een oorzaak van obstipatie. Ned Tijdschr Geneesk 129: 1624–167.

17. Preston DM, Lennard-Jones JE, Thomas BM. 1984. The balloon proctogram. Br J Surg 71: 29–32.

18. Broden B, Snellman B. 1968. Procidentia of the rectum studied with cineradiography. Dis Colon Rectum 11: 330–347.

19. Hoffman MJ, Kodner IJ, Fry RD. 1984. Internal intussusception of the rectum. Diagnosis and surgical management. Dis Colon Rectum 27: 435–441.

20. Bartolo DCC, Roe AM, Virjee I, McCMortensen NJ. 1985. Evacuation proctography in obstructed defaecation and rectal intussusception. Br J Surg 72: S111–S116.

21. Kuijpers JHC, de Morree HH. 1986. Intussusceptie van het rectum: fantasie of werkelijkheid? Ned Tijdschr Geneesk 13: 590–592.

22. Ihre T. 1972. Internal procidentia of the rectum: treatment and results. Scand J Gastroenterol 7: 643–646.

23. Goldberg SM, Gordon PH, Nivatvongs S. 1980. Essentials of ano-rectal surgery. First ed. Philadelphia: JB Lippincott.

24. Berman JR, Manning DH, Dudley-Wright KRn. 1985. Anatomic specificity in the diagnosis and treatment of internal rectal prolapse. Dis Colon Rectum 28: 816–826.

25. Bentley JFR. 1964. Some new observations on megacolon in infancy and childhood with special reference to the management of megasigmoid and megarectum. Dis Colon Rectum 7: 462–470.

26. Ehrenpreis T. 1967. Megacolon and megarectum in older children and young adults. Classification and Terminology. Proc Roy Soc Med 60: 799–801.

27. Duhamel B. 1966. Histological investigations into idiopathic megacolon. Arch Dis Child 41: 150–154.

28. Thomas CG, Bream CA, DeConnick P. 1970. Posterior sphincterotomy and rectal myotomy in the management of Hirschsprung's disease. Ann Surg 171: 796–810.

29. Nissen S, Bar-Maor JA, Levy E. 1969. Ano-rectal myomectomy in the treatment of short segment Hirschsprung's disease. Ann Surg 170: 969–977.

30. Lynn HB, van Heerden JA. 1975. Rectal myectomy in Hirschsprung's disease. A decade of experience. Arch Surg 110: 991–994.

31. Clayden GS, Lawson JON. 1976. Investigation and management of long-standing chronic constipation in childhood. Arch Dis Child 51: 918–923.

32. McCready RA, Beart RW. 1980. Adult Hirschsprung's disease. Results of surgical treatment of Mayo Clinic. Dis Colon Rectum 23: 401–407.

33. Shandling B, Desjardins JG. 1969. Anal myomectomy for constipation. J Ped Surg 4: 115–118.

34. Martelli H, Devroede G, Arhan P, Dyguay C. 1978. Mechanisms of idiopathic constipation: outlet obstruction. Gastroenterology 75: 623–631

35. Marks MM. 1967. The rectal side of the rectocele. Dis Colon Rectum 10: 387–388.

36. Sehapayak S. 1985. Trans-rectal repair of rectocele: An extended armentarium of colorectal surgeons. A report of 355 cases. Dis Colon Rectum 28: 422–433.

37. Capps WF. 1975. Rectoplasty and perineoplasty for the symptomatic rectocele. A report of fifty cases. Dis Colon Rectum 18: 237–243.

38. Sullivan ES, Leaverton GH, Hardwick CE. 1968. Trans-rectal perineal repair: an adjunct to improved function after ano-rectal surgery. Dis Colon Rectum 11: 106–114.

3. Faecal incontinence

3.1 Neurological causes

M. SWASH

Introduction

Incontinence is a common affliction, particularly in the elderly. The term incontinence is often used to refer only to urinary incontinence because the latter is generally regarded as a more common disorder than faecal incontinence, or than double incontinence. However, it is very likely that the frequency of faecal incontinence has been under-estimated [1]. For example, among elderly hospitalised populations faecal incontinence is a factor leading to disability in nearly half the population surveyed, and Leigh and Turnberg [2] found that more than half of the patients presenting to their medical gastroenterology clinic with the complaint of diarrhoea were, in reality, incontinent of faeces. Similary, incontinence, both of urine and faeces, is frequently not pursued by neurologists thus leaving the patient to deal with the problem as best he or she can. This lack of medical awareness of the frequency and severity of incontinence is, perhaps, an understandable reaction to the relative ineffectiveness of therapy, particularly when there is a neurological cause.

Neurological causes of incontinence usually affect both the ano-rectal and bladder sphincter systems since these two sets of neurones and their connections are closely related both anatomically and functionally. In this review emphasis will be placed on faecal incontinence, but the relationship of this disorder to urinary incontinence will be stressed where relevant.

Classification of neurological causes of incontinence

Much controversy has been engendered in attempts to classify urinary incontinence in terms of functional disturbances attributed to lesions at various levels in the nervous system but faecal incontinence has not, hitherto, been considered in these terms. Nonetheless, it is well known that urinary and faecal incontinence develop in patients with lesions in the brain or brain stem, with

spinal cord lesions, and with damage to the pelvic, autonomic, or somatic innervation of the smooth and striated sphincter musculature controlling the voiding of urine and faeces. It is therefore common usage to refer to upper and lower motor neuron lesions with respect to the bladder so that the term 'spastic bladder' is in common use. However, true spasticity in the neurological sense does not occur in the smooth detrusor muscle of the dome of the bladder since this muscle is not innervated by somatic efferent neurons, and there are no muscle spindles in the smooth musculature. The term 'spastic bladder' is therefore illogical and it is this illogicality that has led to much difficulty in the understanding of the functional deficit found in cystometrograms. Hald and Bradley have attempted to relate the different clinical and cystometric varieties of urinary incontinence to a neuro-anatomical classification dependent on four neural loops [3]. These loops consist of:
- a frontal lobe to brain stem system,
- a brain stem to sacral detrusor nucleus system,
- a detrusor to pudendal nucleus system (an intrasacral loop) and
- a frontal lobe to sacral pudendal nucleus neuronal system.

Evidence for the existence of these discrete functional systems is incomplete and the chief attraction of this concept of control of the urinary bladder is that it can be loosely related to the older concept of an uninhibited or reflex bladder, corresponding to lesions in the frontal lobe brain stem connections, or brain stem detrusor nucleus connections, and to the sensory or motor paralytic bladders that correspond to more distal lesions. In addition, the more rostral lesions are said to correspond to failure to store urine and the more caudal to failure to empty the bladder. Clearly, these functional concepts, linked only loosely to anatomical theories, do not provide a ready approach to understanding the differing roles of the autonomic and somatic nervous systems in the control of the bladder in clinical practice. In the present state of knowledge it is probably best to regard these systems as inextricably inter-related, and simply to accept that understanding of how they inter-relate functionally in everyday life is incomplete.

However, similar concepts can be applied to understanding the control mechanisms of faecal incontinence and defaecation. Normal ano-rectal continence implies the ability to store faeces and to expel faecal matter at socially convenient times. There must therefore exist an ability to *inhibit* reflexly-induced defaecation, and to *induce* defaecation either voluntarily, or by allowing enhancement of ongoing levels of reflex excitation at the appropriate time. It is a commonplace observation that there are at least three normal patterns of defaecation. For example defaecation may occur in response to internal drives, as in the defaecatory desire that commonly occurs after a large meal. Defaecation also occurs as a time-locked phenomenon, for example the defaecation that ordinarily occurs shortly after rising in the morning (and which is so evident in the jet-lagged traveller) and defaecation can occur as a voluntary act, apparently irrespective of the previous two factors. It is thus evident that both the somatic efferent and afferent nervous systems, and the autonomic innervation of the smooth muscle are under voluntary control in so far as these two muscular systems are responsible for continence of faeces. Most descriptions of normal defaecation commence with increasing filling and pressure within the rectum by the transit of faeces from colon to rectum. This leads experimentally to progressive relaxation of the internal anal sphincter, and the recruitment of the voluntary act of defaecation by elevation of pelvic floor, contraction of abdominal and diaphragm muscles, and relaxation of puborectalis and of external anal sphincter muscles [4–6]. The deleterious effects, if any, of parasympathetic lesions on this process are uncertain and it is not known whether colonic or rectal contraction occurs in defaecation.

In considering the causes of faecal incontinence both functional factors within the bowel, age, degree of incontinence, and lesions in the ano-rectum, its musculature, its nerve supply, and the central control mechanisms must be considered. In addition, there is evidence that vascular factors, particularly those that interfere with the natural engorgement of the anal cushions, may be important. The classification evolved in our work at St. Mark's is given in the table.

Neurological causes of incontinence

Lesions of the central control system in the brain, brain stem and spinal cord rostral to the sacral nucleus of Onuf are conventionally termed upper motor neuron lesions. Thus any disease process that has resulted in functionally important damage to descending and ascending pathways concerned with defaecation can cause incontinence.

It has long been known that voluntary control of the bladder and rectum is represented in the cerebral cortex. Indeed, Kleist indicated that the bladder and rectum were represented both in motor and sensory cortex on the medial surface of the hemisphere [7], a view endorsed by Förster. Subsequently, Penfield and Rasmussen were able to obtain sensations of bladder and rectal fullness by stimulation of the cortex a little more superiorly on the medial surface of the hemisphere [8]. However, lesions at this discrete site have not been reported as leading to disorders of defaecation or micturition. Frontal lobe disorders, nonetheless, particularly in patients with lesions of the medial and inferior surfaces of the frontal lobes, are well known causes of incontinence. Thus meningiomas arising from the falx cerebri, or from the olefactory groove, that impinge upon the medial or inferior surfaces of the frontal cortex may present with incontinence. In these patients incontinence often consists of

112

Table 1. Classification of the causes of faecal incontinence.*

A. *Normal sphincters and pelvic floor*
    Diarrhoea:
        Infective
        Inflammatory bowel disease
        Intestinal resection
        Metabolic (e.g. diabetes mellitus)
    Fistula/colostomy

B. *Abnormal function of sphincters and/or pelvic floor*
    Partial incontinence:
        Internal sphincter deficiency:
            Previous surgery (e.g. anal stretch, sphincterotomy)
            Rectal prolapse
            Third-degree haemorrhoids
        Faecal impaction:
            The elderly
            Generalised neurological disorders (e.g. mental defect)
        Minor external sphincter and pelvic floor denervation
    Major incontinence:
        Congenital anomalies of the ano-rectum
        Trauma:
            Iatrogenic
            Obstetric
            Fractures of pelvis
            Impalement
        Complete rectal prolapse
        Rectal carcinoma
        Ano-rectal infection (e.g. lymphogranuloma)
        Idiopathic (primary neurogenic faecal incontinence)
        Drug intoxication (especially in the elderly)
        Neurological:
            Upper motor-neuron lesion:
                Cerebral:
                    multiple strokes
                    metastases and other tumours
                    dementia and other degenerative disorders
                    trauma
                    multiple sclerosis
                Spinal:
                    multiple sclerosis
                    metastases and other tumours
                    degenerative diseases (e.g. B_{12} deficiency)
            Lower motor-neuron lesion:
                Cauda equina (tumour or trauma)
                Peripheral neuropathy (diabetes)
                Tabes dorsalis
                Lumbar meningomyelocele (spina bifida)

---

* From Henry and Swash (.14).

defaecation or micturition at inappropriate times and in inappropriate places rather than frank urge incontinence.

Incontinence may also be a presenting feature in patients with decompensated hydrocephalus. In the latter patients there is no evidence of functional disturbance of cortical neuronal function and the incontinence must result from damage to the descending pathways between the cortex and the brain stem by the expanding ventricular system. For anatomical reasons the corticomotor pathway from the medial surface of the hemisphere is more likely to be stretched and deformed by the expanding lateral ventricles than is the corticomotor pathway from the lateral convexity of the cortex. Thus these patients commonly also present with an apractic gait disorder, and may be found to have brisk reflexes in the legs and extensor plantar responses whereas motor function in the arms and in the bulbar muscles is spared. Incontinence, gait apraxia, and extensor plantar responses are thus features of decompensated hydrocephalus [9]. In degenerative diseases, particularly Alzheimer dementia and multifocal cerebrovascular disease, the lesions responsible for incontinence are of necessity uncertain. In brainstem vascular disease, incontinence is not usually a major problem unless there is pseudobulbar palsy with the typical pseudobulbar disturbance of affect. However, pontine lesions may result in incontinence. Similarly, incontinence of urine or faeces in multiple sclerosis can be correlated most closely with the development of lesions in the bifrontal white matter rather than with brain stem disease. Brain stem mechanisms for control of ano-rectal function are, at present, controversial but there is increasing evidence for major representation of smooth muscle innervation, important for the control of normal gut motility, in the nuclei of the dorsal nucleus of the vagus, and in the locus coeruleus.

In spinal cord lesions there is loss of supranuclear control of the sacral centres for defaecation and micturition so that in the absence of obstruction to micturition or defaecation or of infection an automatic pattern of micturition and defaecation may be established. However, the absence of normal afferent information as to the degree of filling of the ano-rectum and colon, and of the bladder often results in distension, overfilling and injury to these organs with consequent secondary effects of a profound nature. These include loss of viscoelasticity of the wall of the ano-rectum, loss of the normal smooth muscle responses to filling and inflation and thus abnormal compliance and incontinence. Thus there is not only loss of the normal functions of micturition and defaecation, but loss of the normal storage function for urine and faeces in these patients. Nathan and Smith [10, 11] demonstrated the location of the afferent and efferent pathways for micturition in the human spinal cord but there is no such definite information for the pathways subserving defaecation although they are presumed to be close to those related to micturition. The processes of micturition and defaecation are, nonetheless, separate in functional terms; it is difficult, if not impossible, to micturate and defaecate at the same time.

Lower motor neuron lesions

Damage to the somatic afferent and efferent pathway to the ano-rectum results from lesions in the lumbosacral spine, for example cauda equina disease [12] due to spondylosis, tumour, sacral meningomyelocele, or trauma. It may also occur with intrapelvic disease involving the sacral plexus, particularly trauma or metastases, with peripheral neuropathy, particularly diabetes mellitus, tabes dorsalis, or after trauma to the pudendal and perineal nerves. Of these the two most common factors are idiopathic damage to the pudendal and perineal innervations of the pelvic sphincter musculature, and spondylotic damage to the cauda equina. In addition, in women, significant damage can occur during childbirth to the pudendal and perineal innervations of the external anal sphincter and periurethral striated sphincter muscles respectively, and to the pelvic innervation (direct somatic S2 motor branches) of the puborectalis and of the intramural fibres of the striated urethral sphincter fibres [13, 14].

In patients with stress urinary incontinence there is damage to the periurethral striated sphincter musculature, usually related to injury to this innervation during childbirth [15]. Similarly, in idiopathic neurogenic faecal incontinence there is damage to both the pudendal and direct pelvic innervations of the external anal sphincter and puborectalis muscles respectively. The latter results in loss of the ano-rectal angulation, from weakness of the puborectalis muscle, and so to defaecation during abdominal straining, coughing, sneezing or twisting movements. The latter, although initiated by obstetric trauma, deteriorates as a result of ageing, the development of co-existent spondylosis with cauda equina disease, or stretch-induced damage to these innervations during perineal descent associated with straining at stool [14]. Similar damage, occasionally severe enough to result in incontinence, may occur in patients with a long history of intractable straining and constipation, although this is an unusual cause of the development of faecal incontinence. Some of these relationships are illustrated in Figure 7 in chapter 1.2.

Sensory disturbances

Damage to the innervation of these muscles would be expected to result also in abnormalities in sensory function within the ano-rectum. These are commonly present, although not stressed in clinical examination. Most patients with faecal incontinence have difficulty differentiating faeces from flatus and many are often unaware that they have been incontinent until they discover that their underclothes are soiled. In tabes dorsalis incontinence may be prominent, but this probably results from a combination of sensory disturbance and autonomic damage. It appears likely that damage to the smooth muscle of the intrinsic sphincter system alone does not result in incontinence to formed stool although there may be difficulties in the perception of filling of the ano-rectum, particularly when the faeces are liquid, or when the ano-rectum is filled with flatus rather than faeces. Thus the smooth musculature may be important in maintaining apposition of the mucosal walls of the viscus and so in maintaining a normal sensory system. However, the precise functional inter-relationships of the smooth muscle sphincters with the striated sphincter musculature of the pelvic floor is, at present, uncertain.

References

1. Thomas TM, Egan M, Walgrove A, Meade TW. 1984. The prevalence of faecal and double incontinence. Community Med 6: 216–220.
2. Leigh RJ, Turnberg LA. 1982. Faecal incontinence; the unvoiced symptom. Lancet 1: 1349–1351.
3. Hald T, Bradley WE. 1982. The Urinary Bladder; neurology and dynamics. William and Wilkins, Baltimore, London: 22–57.
4. Baldi F, Ferrarine F, Corinaldesi R et al. 1982. Function of the internal anal sphincter and rectal sensitivity in idiopathic constipation. Digestion 24: 14–22.
5. Parks AG, Porter NH, Nelzack J. 1962. Experimental studies of the reflex mechanisms controlling the muscles of the pelvic floor. Dis Colon Rectum 5: 407–414.
6. Phillips SF, Edwards DAW. 1965. Some aspects of anal continence and defaecation. Gut 6: 396–406.
7. Kleist K. 1922/1934. Kriegsverletzungen des Gehirns. In: Handbuch der Ärztlichen Erfahrungen im Weltkriege 1914/1918. Band IV: Geistes- und Nervenkrankheiten. Bonhoeffer K. ed. Leipzig Verlag: 343–1369.
8. Penfield W, Rasmussen T. 1950. The Cerebral Cortex of Man. Macmillan-New York.
9. Hakim S, Adams RD. 1965. The special clinical problem of symptomatic hydrocephalus with normal corticospinal fluid pressure. J Neurol Sci 2: 307–315.
10. Nathan PW, Smith MC. 1951. The centripetal pathway from the bladder and urethra within the spinal cord. J Neurol Neurosurg Psychiatry 14: 262–289.
11. Nathan PW, Smith MC. 1958. The centrifugal pathway for micturition within the spinal cord. J Neurol Neurosurg Psychiatry 21: 177–189.
12. Swash M, Snooks SJ. 1986. Slowed motor conduction in lumbosacral nerve roots in cauda equina lesions. J Neurol Neurosurg Psychiatry 49: 808–816.
13. Snooks SJ, Swash M, Setchell M, Henry MM. 1984. Injury to innervation of the pelvic floor sphincter musculature in childbirth. Lancet 2: 546–550.
14. In Henry MM, Swash M. (eds) 1985. Coloproctology and the Pelvic Floor. Butterworths, London: 222–228.
15. Snooks SJ, Badenoch D, Tiptaft R, Swash M. 1985. Perineal nerve damage in genuine stress urinary incontinence: an electrophysiological study. Br J Urol 57: 422–426.

3.2 Obstetric causes

M.M. HENRY, S.J. SNOOKS, M. SWASH & M. SETCHELL

Introduction

Faecal incontinence occurs predominantly in women in whom as many as 60% report a history of preceding problems with childbirth [1]. The possibility that pelvic floor damage may be incurred during parturition was raised at the beginning of the century by Hertz [2] but this has been largely ignored since. Obstetric injury may clearly give rise to loss of ano-rectal function in cases where there has been direct damage to the anal sphincter ring (e.g., third degree perineal tears). However, the majority of women who develop faecal incontinence do not have a history suggestive of such an injury. Hence other factors must be relevant to the development of faecal incontinence particularly in view of the fact that the external anal sphincter ring is not considered to be of fundamental significance to gross continence. The puborectalis muscle is generally considered to be the principal factor responsible for ano-rectal continence [3]. Another factor which has to be considered is that perhaps the pregnancy itself rather than transmission of the foetal head through the birth canal may be responsible for pelvic floor weakness. This could arise secondarily to the effect of relaxing on supporting tissues in the pelvis or be an effect on levator musculature caused by raised intra-abdominal pressure, for example.

Indirect evidence of denervation in the pelvic floor musculature was found in 80% of patients with faecal incontinence investigated by enzyme histochemical techniques applied to a series of biopsies from the pelvic floor [1]. Further support for the theory that faecal incontinence in many patients was a consequence of denervation was obtained by single fibre EMG studies of the external anal sphincter muscle [4]. Demonstration of delay in the transmission of an electrical stimulus along the pudendal nerves strongly suggested that a peripheral nerve injury was responsible for the neuropathy in most patients [5].

The aetiology of the nerve damage has been the subject of considerable debate and interest. Clearly some patients develop neuronal damage as part of a generalised neurological disease (e.g., disseminated sclerosis) or local neurological disease (e.g., the peripheral neuropathy associated with diabetes mellitus or alcoholism). In our experience of managing pelvic floor disorders at St. Mark's Hospital, London, these conditions are rare.

Since the initial description of the descending perineum syndrome [6] it has been recognised that there is a group of patients who habitually strain at defaecation and who on examination are found to have abnormal descent of the pelvic floor. Many of these patients have pelvic floor denervation and suffer from faecal incontinence [7]. The possibility exists that the denervation in these patients arises secondary to a stretch injury to the nerves supplying the pelvic floor. Alternatively it is equally possible that the denervation is the primary process with pelvic floor descent occurring as a secondary event which may then compound the neuropathy.

As discussed above, most women with ano-rectal incontinence present with a history of problems with childbirth which may preceed the onset of incontinence by a period varying from several months to several years [8]. It is possible, therefore, that in these women neurogenic damage is induced by compression of the pudendal nerves which are situated on the side wall of the pelvis by the passage of the foetal head.

This theory has been investigated in a group of women, 51 of which were studied both before and after delivery, and a further 71 women who were studied after delivery only.

Patients

One hundred and twenty-two pregnant women (62 primigravidae and 60 multiparae) aged 16-39 years (mean age 28 years) consecutively referred to the Obstetric Unit at St. Bartholomew's Hospital, London were studied. None of these women had a history of previous injury to the external anal sphincter muscle and none was diabetic or suffered from neurological disease. One hundred and two women were delivered vaginally (mean birth weight 3.3 ± 0.5 Kg), 70 without forceps assistance and 32 with the application of Simpsons' forceps. Thirty-one women had elective epidural anaesthesia and episiotomy had been performed in 58. Twenty women, including 11 primigravidae, had elective Caesarean sections for pelvic disproportion. All 122 women delivered live healthy babies.

Thirty-four nulliparous women served as controls. All had a normal defaecatory pattern and none suffered from metabolic or neurological disease.

Methods

Perineal position and descent

Measurements of the plane of the perineum in relationship to the plane of the bony outlet of the pelvis were made using a device previously described [7]. Measurements were made during straining and in the resting state in the group of 71 women studied exclusively after delivery. Measurements were made in the period 48–72 hours and repeated at 2 months after delivery.

Pudendal nerve terminal motor latency (PNTML)

This method was developed at St.Mark's Hospital, London from the technique of electro-ejaculation described by Brindley [9]. The stimulating device comprises a rubber finger stall with 2 metal stimulating electrodes at the tip and 2 metal surface electrodes at the base of the glove. The finger stall is inserted into the anal canal and the tip brought into contact with the pudendal nerve on each side at the level of the ischial spine. Electrical stimuli of the order of 50V and 0.1 mS are delivered and the latency between the onset of the stimulus and contraction of the external anal sphincter (detected by the surface electrodes) is measured.

Recordings were made in patients only after delivery; it was considered unethical to stimulate the pelvic floor prior to delivery.

Single fibre EMG

Single fibre EMG of the external anal sphincter muscle was measured using the technique previously described from this laboratory [4]. The mean number of single muscle fibre action potentials recorded in 20 different positions, through 4 separate skin insertions, is called the fibre density (FD) and represents an index of the mean number of muscle fibres innervated by one motor unit within the uptake of the electrode [10].

Studies were performed in patients prior to delivery and repeated at 2 months after delivery.

Statistical methods

The Wilcoxon Rank Sum Test for paired and unpaired data was used for comparison between groups.

120

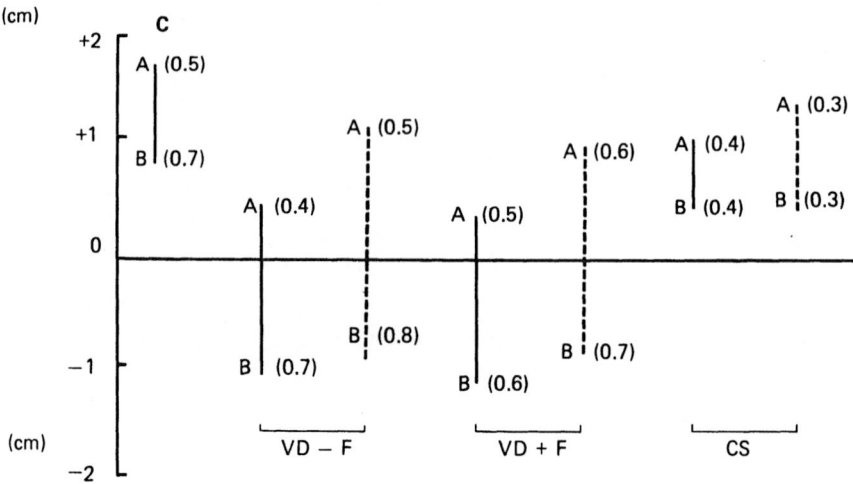

Figure 1. Perineal planes in relationship to plane of ischial tuberosities. Plane of ischial tuberosities represented by horizontal unbroken line. Figures below line hence represent descent of the perineum below this level. (A) at rest (B) on straining. Unbroken vertical lines: 48–72h after delivery or in controls. Broken vertical lines: 2 months after delivery. C: control; VD: Vaginal Delivery; F: Forceps; CS: Caesarean Section.

Results

Perineal measurements

These results are displayed in Figure 1. There was significant descent of the plane of the perineum at rest and during straining in the group of women delivered vaginally when measured at 48–72 hours after delivery. When repeated at 2 months there was significant descent during straining alone in this group compared with controls. Those women who underwent Caesarean section had perineal positions similar to the control group.

PNTML and FD measurements

These results are displayed in Table 1. The FD was significantly increased in the external anal sphincter muscle from a value of 1.4 in the ante-natal period to 1.6 at 2 months after delivery ($p<0.01$) There was no change in FD in the ante-natal and post-natal studies in the 6 women delivered by Caesarean section. The FD in these women was similar to that obtained in the control subjects.

Obstetric factors and relationship to pelvic floor neuropathy

A variety of factors were assessed by multifactorial analysis to determine which, if any, were positively correlated with the development of neuropathic damage.

Parity

Analysis of the ante-natal results demonstrated that the FD in the external anal sphincter muscle in multiparae was increased (*p*<0.01) compared with both primigravidae and control subjects. In the postnatal period the FD in multiparae was greater than in primigravidae (*p*<0.01).

Forceps

In primigravidae delivered with forceps the PNTML at 48–72 hours and the FD 2 months after delivery were increased (*p*<0.01) compared with primigravidae delivered without forceps.

There were 20 multiparous women who had had forceps delivery, each was paired with a multiparous woman who did not have forceps but in whom parity and duration of the second stage of labour was the same. The PNTML at 48–72

Table 1. Fibre density, pudendal latency: effect of parity and forceps delivery.

Group		FD(SD)	PNTML (SD) (ms)	*n*
Controls			1.9 (0.2)	24
		1.37 (0.09)		34
Vag. P	(A)	1.31 (0.06)	(P1) 2.1 (0.4)[a]	25
	(P2)	1.41 (0.08)	(P2) 1.9 (0.2)	19
Vag. P + F	(A)	1.34 (0.05)	(P1) 2.4 (0.4)[a]	25
	(P2)	1.58 (0.12)[a]	(P2) 2.0 (0.2)	21
Vag. M	(A)	1.44 (0.16)[b]	(P1) 2.3 (0.4)[a]	45
	(P2)	1.67 (0.18)[a]	(P2) 2.1 (0.3)	38
Vag. M + F	(A)	–	(P1) 2.4 (0.4)[a]	7
	(P2)	–	(P2) 2.1 (0.3)	7

A: ante-natal; P1 and P2: postnatal at 48–72h and 2 months; Vag: vaginal delivery; P: primigravidae; M: multigravidae; F: forceps; FD: fibre density; PNTML: pudendal nerve terminal motor latency.

[a] *p*<0.01 difference from control or ante-natal groups.
[b] *p*<0.01 difference from primigravidae ante-natal group.

hours was greater in women delivered with forceps than in those delivered without forceps ($p<0.02$).

Duration of second stage of labour

Ten multiparous women with a duration of the second stage of labour of less than 0.5 hours were matched with 10 multiparous women whose labour was greater than 0.5 hours. The PNTML at 48–72 hours after delivery in the long duration group was greater than in the short duration group.

Epidural anaesthesia

No differences were found in the PNTML and FD in patients having forceps assisted deliveries in a group of women who had epidural anaesthesia compared to a group who had forceps delivery without epidural anaesthesia.

Perineal trauma

Three groups were compared: episiotomy alone, perineal tear and no perineal tear (Table 2). The PNTML 48–72 hours after delivery and FD 2 months after delivery were increased in each group compared with control subjects ($p<0.01$). Four women sustained third degree perineal tears, three of these had a marked increase in PNTML 48–72 hours after delivery and all 4 had an increased FD 2 months after delivery.

Table 2. Perineal trauma.

Group	FD (SD) (2 months)	PNTML (SD) (ms) 48–72 h postnatal	n
E	1.56 (0.27)[a]	2.2 (0.3)[a]	21
T (1, 2)	1.56 (0.21)[a]	2.3 (0.4)[a]	23
T (3)	2.10 (0.24)[a]	2.8 (0.4)[a]	4
No T	1.54 (0.16)[a]	2.2 (0.4)[a]	21
Controls		1.9 (0.2)	24
	1.37 (0.09)		34

E: episiotomy; T (1, 2, 3): 1st, 2nd, 3rd degree perineal tear.
[a] $p<0.01$ difference from controls.

Birth weight

There was a significant linear correlation between the PNTML 48–72 hours after delivery and birth weight (r = 0.4, $p<0.01$).

Head circumference

No correlation was demonstrated between head circumference and PNTML.

Discussion

We have demonstrated that vaginal delivery and not the pregnancy itself is responsible for damage to the nerve supply of the pelvic floor as evidenced by an overall increase in the PNTML and FD in those patients delivered vaginally. These changes were not observed in those patients delivered by Caesarean section. An increase in PNTML implies damage to or loss of a population of rapidly conducting, large, myelinated motor fibres in the distal portion of the nerve or a conduction block as a consequence of damage to those motor fibres between the point of stimulation and the muscle itself.

Multiparae displayed evidence of denervation in the ante-natal period as demonstrated by a raised FD compared with the nulliparous controls. Multiparae also had a more markedly increased PNTML after vaginal delivery than primigravidae. Hence, parity is an important factor in the development of neurogenic damage.

Similarly, the application of forceps seemed to be responsible for increased risk of damage to the pudendal nerves during delivery. In women delivered by forceps the duration of second stage of labour was also a factor associated with nerve damage. A third degree perineal tear was associated with a severe neurogenic injury, independent of whether or not forceps had been applied. In contrast, the employment of an episiotomy or epidural anaesthesia were not found to be positively correlated factors.

The most likely explanation for pudendal nerve damage after vaginal delivery is that these nerves sustain a combination of direct injury in the pelvis and a traction injury during elongation of the birth canal during delivery. In 60% of women this injury is reversible [11]. These observations suggest that although the damage to the pelvic floor is unrecognisable at the time, it is common and may be responsible for serious problems in the future.

Identification of risk factors may ultimately be of considerable value to the practice of obstetrics such that, hopefully, faecal incontinence may become increasingly less common in succeeding generations of women.

124

Acknowledgements

We are most grateful to the medical and nursing staff of the Obstetric Unit at St. Bartholomew's Hospital, London for their kind assistance in this study. Financial support was provided by The Royal College of Surgeons of England and by the St. Mark's Hospital Research Foundation.

References

1. Parks AG, Swash M, Urich H. 1977. Sphincter denervation in ano-rectal incontinence and rectal prolapse. Gut 18: 656–665.
2. Hertz AF. 1909. Constipation and Allied Disorders. Oxford University Press, London, pp 110–113.
3. Hardcastle JD, Parks AG. 1970. A study of anal incontinence and some principles of surgical treatment. Proc Roy Soc Med 63 (suppl): 116–118.
4. Neill ME, Swash M. 1980. Increased motor unit fibre density in the external anal sphincter muscle in ano-rectal incontinence: a single fibre EMG study. J Neurol Neurosurg and Psych 43: 343–347.
5. Kiff ES, Swash M. 1984. Slowed conduction in the pudendal nerves in idiopathic (neurogenic) faecal incontinence. Br J Surg 71: 614–616.
6. Parks AG, Porter NH, Hardcastle JD. 1966. The syndrome of the descending perineum. Proc Roy Soc Med 59: 477–482.
7. Henry MM, Parks AG, Swash M. 1982. The pelvic floor musculature in the descending perineum syndrome. Br J Surg 69: 470–472.
8. Henry MM, Parks AG, Swash M. 1980. An electrophysiological study of the anal reflex in patients with idiopathic faecal incontinence. Br J Surg 67: 781–783.
9. Brindley GA. 1981. Electro-ejaculation: its technique, neurological implications and uses. J Neurol Neurosurg Psych 44: 9–18.
10. Stalberg E, Thiele B. 1975. Motor unit fibre density in the extensor digitorum communis muscle. J Neurol Neurosurg and Psych 38: 874–880.
11. Snooks SJ, Swash M, Henry MM, Setchell M. 1984. Injury to innervation of pelvic floor musculature in childbirth. Lancet ii: 546–550.

3.3 Iatrogenic causes

M.R.B. KEIGHLEY

Introduction

Faecal incontinence is not a diagnosis but a symptom and one which is much more common than is often realised by many general practitioners. Patients are extremely embarrassed about their symptoms and refuse to speak about the problem. Many become recluse, having lost all feelings of self respect. Many patients are frightened to speak to their doctor about their symptoms for fear of being misunderstood. For this reason it is unlikely that the true incidence of this symptom will be fully realised until the medical profession are prepared to ask direct questions of patients with proctological symptoms [1].

Iatrogenic causes

Faecal incontinence may be due to a variety of disorders. The underlying disorders of patients who gave a history of incontinence of liquid and solid faeces occurring more than twice a year between 1975 and 1980 were recorded (Table 1). A high proportion of these patients had a carcinoma of the rectum or inflammatory bowel disease. A smaller number had had a previous operation on the colon and rectum. Rectal prolapse was an important cause, as were previous operations on the anal canal. It is this group of patients who have had previous operations that deserves our closest attention since they are surgical catastrophes. They represent iatrogenic incontinence and are those which could easily be avoided by careful assessment and appropriate operative surgery. Over the past ten years (1975–1985) 237 patients with faecal incontinence have been referred. The causes of incontinence are listed in Table 2. Although obstetric trauma and pelvic floor neuropathy without a history of obstetric injury were two common groups, sphincter injury from previous surgical therapy was, in our experience, the most common group of subjects presenting with incontinence. Details of the 57 patients with sphincter injury are shown on Table 2.

Trauma

In addition there were 5 patients who had undergone severe perineal trauma after road traffic accidents, where the sphincter had been injured in association with urethral damage and fractures to the pelvis and the femur. In these cases an initial proximal colostomy has been raised and subsequent manometric studies had revealed complete loss of sphincter over a segment of the anal canal. In each case the sphincter defect was reconstituted as a flapover repair and a proximal colostomy was not disturbed. Subsequent closure of the colostomy was associated with complete return of continence in all five cases.

Anal dilatation

Sixteen patients were rendered incontinent after anal dilatation. In 15 of the 16 cases a repeated anal dilatation had been performed and in many of these patients there was very little evidence of anal pathology. Although the history was commonly one of anal discomfort associated with haemorrhoids, or with

Table 1. Underlying diagnosis in 346 patients with incontinence seen by the author between 1975–1980.

Diagnosis		No. of patients
Carcinoma of the rectum		104
Villous papilloma		14
Inflammatory bowel disease		70
Ulcerative colitis	21	
Crohn's disease	37	
Diverticular disease	10	
Radiation proctitis	2	
Previous colo-rectal operation		32
Ileo-rectal anastomosis		
for inflammatory bowel disease	14	
Low anterior resection	12	
Colo-anal anastomosis	6	
Rectal prolapse		40
Descending perineum syndrome		22
Previous operation on the anal canal		20
Trauma following road accident		3
Obstetric trauma		5
Repeated self dilatation		4
Imperforate anus		3
Neurological		5
Bolus obstruction		16
Cause unknown		8

an anal fissure, objective evidence of the presence of actual anal pathology was lacking in 7 of 12 cases. Subsequent examination of the 16 patients who had undergone anal dilatation and who had become incontinent revealed that 9 of them had gross perineal descent during straining. It has been suggested that some of these patients may never have had any evidence of haemorrhoids or fissure but because patients continued to complain of anal discomfort, dilatation was repeated without there being any obvious intra-anal pathology. In such patients the pelvic floor was commonly severely damaged. In some patients there was no anal pathology but the patient presented with gross perineal descent at rest or during straining. In these patients there is often inherent weakness of the pelvic floor and many of the patients are rendered completely incontinent by forceful anal dilatation. It is now our policy never to perform an anal dilatation in female patients when there is evidence of perineal descent at rest or during straining. Furthermore, we never repeat anal dilatation irrespective of the presence of pathology for fear of rendering patients incontinent. Anal dilatation is associated with a profound fall in

Table 2. Aetiology of incontinence in 237 patients being considered for surgical treatment. (Patients with malignancy, active ulcerative colitis and rectal prolapse excluded).

			Perineal descent
Descending perineum syndrome alone		36	(36)
Idiopathic pelvic floor neuropathy		15	(–)
Previous successful rectopexy but persistent incontinence		25	(15)
Surgical trauma		57	(15)
Anal dilatation	16		(9)
Subcutaneous sphincterotomy	6		(–)
Laying open fistula in ano	24		(4)
Haemorrhoidectomy	5		(2)
Excision of fissure	2		(–)
Trauma following road accident		5	
Obstetric trauma		32	(20)
Repeated self dilatation		6	
Imperforate anus		6	
Neurological		22	(2)
Multiple sclerosis	3		(–)
Von Recklinghausen's disease	2		(–)
Diabetes mellitus	8		(2)
Central prolapsed disc	4		(–)
Sacral involvement in a pelvic neoplasm	3		(–)
Metastases in dorsal or cervical spine	2		(–)
Unknown		8	
Faecal impaction		25	(–)

resting anal canal pressures which may be sustained for over five years [2]. Anal dilatation disrupts the fibres not only of the internal sphincter but of the external sphincter and pelvic floor as well [3]. It is hardly to be surprising therefore that this procedure is associated with some incontinence. Indeed, flatus incontinence is remarkably common but usually does not persist. Use of the Park's intra-anal retractor may have a similar effect. We have preliminary evidence that the use of this device is associated with a reduction in resting anal pressure of about 20 cm water 6–12 months after operation. Interestingly, many of these patients also complain of incontinence of flatus initially. These and other observations indicate that anal dilatation which achieves a similar reduction in anal pressure is potentially dangerous and should be used sparingly [4].

Sphincterotomy

Six patients had a previous lateral subcutaneous sphincterotomy. However, on electromyography and manometry of the anal canal it appeared that part of the external sphincter had been divided as well. Some of these patients present with a defect causing a gutter in the anal canal along which faecal material may seep. Measurement of anal pressure revealed low resting pressures and leakage of liquid on use of the saline infusion test [5]. There were two additional patients in whom an anal fissure had been excised leaving a deep deformity which was associated with incontinence and soiling. There seems little doubt from these and other observations that the internal sphincter is important for maintaining continence. The internal sphincter keeps the anal canal closed and establishes normal resting anal canal pressure. There is no voluntary component to this motor function but there is a constantly elevated anal canal pressure maintained well above the normal intra-rectal pressure which helps to keep the anal canal closed and the patient continent.

Fistula operations

Twenty-four patients have required some form of sphincter reconstruction for fistula surgery, the majority (16) merely presented with soiling necessitating frequent changes of underclothes without true incontinence. There were only 8 patients in this series who actually had episodes of defaecation without knowledge of their doing so. This group of patients were invariably associated with a high fistula in ano which had been laid open some months or years earlier. Most patients with some defect in defaecation after fistula surgery merely soil because part of the internal sphincter has been divided. True incontinence is associated with a segment of the anal ring which is gaping. Incontinence is invariably aggravated by diarrhoea, as well as psychological instability. True incontinence following fistula surgery was invariably associated with deformity created by the previous operation. Almost all cases who had some incontinence reported that they had had multiple operations performed for fistula in ano. Furthermore there was nearly always a history of recurrent sepsis in the peri-anal region. It seems likely that many cases were associated with a high sinus which had been inadvertently opened into the anal canal creating a supra-levator fistula. This is indeed a tragedy since many of these high sinuses can be managed conservatively without recourse to laying the whole track open. Current physiological studies in our institution have revealed a fall in resting anal canal pressure even when low lying anal fistulas are laid open. However, this phenomenon is usually transient and resting anal pressures return to normal after 6–9 months. By contrast, when more than half of the external sphincter is divided for fistula surgery and particularly when the inner fibres of the puborectalis are divided there is a sustained fall in resting anal pressures which may never recover. Saline infusion tests also reveal early leakage of liquids in these patients despite the fact that they are clinically continent.

Haemorrhoidectomy

Finally there were five patients who were rendered incontinent after haemorrhoidectomy. All had had an anal dilatation at the time of their haemorrhoidectomy and it is possible that the anal stretch rather than the haemorrhoidectomy may have been responsible [6]. Incontinence is fortunately rare after haemorrhoidectomy. It may occur if a stenosis develops leading to proximal faecal impaction or if part of the sphincter has been excised at operation. It is probably wise to avoid haemorrhoidectomy in patients with the descending perineum syndrome and if there is any pre-operative history of impaired control of defaecation.

Incontinence after Hartmann operations

Although it is desirable to close a terminal colostomy in a patient who has had a Hartmann procedure for complicated diverticular disease, this does not always result in return of continence. We have reviewed the results of 56 patients who had a Hartmann procedure. Only 37 were either fit enough or had agreed to have their intestinal tract restored. Of these, 7 had required a secondary stoma to protect the intestinal anastomosis, whilst the remainder had a primary anastomosis without a covering colostomy. There was no mortality and 5 of the 7 patients with a proximal stoma eventually had this closed. We have subsequently analysed the functional results in the 35 patients whose Hartmann procedure has been closed. Seven complained of frank incontinence and 12 regularly wear a perineal pad. Measurement of anal canal pressures in these patients reveals that resting anal canal pressures had a mean value of only 43 cm of water with a maximum squeeze pressure of only 67 cm water. There was a fall in anal canal pressure 4–10 weeks after reconstruction which returned to pre-operative levels 4 months later. The mean rectal capacity in these patients 6 months after restoration of intestinal continuity was only 287 cc of air. Although most patients stated that they preferred natural defaecation, many expressed some dissatisfaction about the quality of continence after closure of the stoma.

Incontinence after low anterior resection

During the past five years 57 low anterior resections have been performed for colo-rectal cancer. Incontinence in the immediate post-operative period was rare and only 7 complained of soiling or leakage of faecal material. In all cases this was a transient phenomenon and full continence was restored within 12 months of operation.

Incontinence after colo-anal resection

Twenty-four colo-anal anastomoses either for low rectal cancer were performed, for high recto-vaginal fistula or for radiation damage to the rectum. There was a high incidence of local recurrence after colo-anal excision for cancer, and in all groups the functional results were poor [7]. Sixteen patients complained of some soiling and 10 were frankly incontinent. Although the degree of incontinence did improve during follow up, 8 patients have to wear pads permanently. As a result of these observations we have largely abandoned this operation for colo-rectal cancer and restrict its use merely for patients with recto-vaginal fistulas or severe radiation damage to the rectum.

Incontinence after ileo-anal pouch anastomosis

Of the 28 mucosal proctectomies and ileo-anal pouch anastomoses so far performed, 20 are evaluable with their ileostomy closed. Of these, 4 leak liquid faeces at night time but the remaining patients have extremely good anal function, though diarrhoea with the passage of more than 7 stools a day is a common feature in these patients who have been reconstructed with the J pouch. Nevertheless, stool frequency does improve with time. Our current practice of constructing a 20x20 cm pouch has largely overcome the problem of frequent bowel movement. Furthermore, the use of mucosectomy from above has eliminated the usually observed fall in resting anal pressures and the incidence of soiling post-operatively has also been considerably reduced too.

Treatment

Treatment of iatrogenic causes of faecal incontinence is largely covered in chapter 3.9. Nevertheless it is our policy to perform a sphincter reconstruction in patients where there is damage to the sphincter ring, from fistula surgery, trauma or excision of a fissure in ano. If there is severe persistent incontinence after anal dilatation, it is our usual policy to perform a postanal repair, particularly in female subjects. If these procedures are unsuccessful we would consider a gracilis sling operation but the need for this type of surgery is small.

References

1. Mandelstam DA. 1985. Faecal incontinence: social and economic factors. In: Henry MM, Swash M (eds) Coloproctology and the pelvic floor. London: Butterworths: 217–222.
2. Hancock BD. 1981. The Lord's procedure for haemorrhoids: a prospective anal pressure study. Br J. Surg 68: 729–730.
3. MacIntyre IMC, Balfour TW. 1972. Results of the Lord non-operative treatment for haemorrhoids. Lancet i: 1094–1095.
4. Keighley MRB, Buchanan P, Minervini S, Arabi Y, Alexander-Williams J. 1979. Prospective trials of minor surgical procedures and high fibre diet for haemorrhoids. Br Med J 2: 967–969.
5. Read NW, Haynes WG, Bartolo DCC, Hall J, Read MG, Donelly TC, Johnson AG. 1983. Use of ano-rectal manometry during rectal infusion of saline to investigate sphincter function in incontinent patients. Gastroenterology 85: 105–115.
6. Snooks S, Henry MM, Swash M. 1984. Faecal incontinence after anal dilatation. Br J Surg 71: 617–618.
7. Keighley MRB, Matheson D. 1980. Functional results of rectal excision and endo-anal anastomosis. Br J Surg 67: 757–761.

3.4 The pathophysiology of anal leakage

Introduction

The anal sphincter contracts to prevent faecal matter escaping from the rectum
at inconvenient times and relaxes to permit defaecation when conditions are
appropriate. There are two situations which challenge the continence mechanisms. These are rises in intra-abdominal pressure and rises in rectal pressure
caused by rectal distension or rectal contraction. The threat of both stresses to
continence is much greater if the rectum contains liquids instead of solids.

Stress faecal incontinence

It is commonly taught that during rises in intra-abdominal pressure continence
is maintained by the operation of a flap valve created by the mobile anterior
rectal wall sealing the top of the anal canal [1]. An alternative mechanism is
that the rises in intra-abdominal pressure compress the upper anal canal above
the level of the pelvic diaphragm creating a flutter valve [2]. Both hypotheses
are mechanically unsound. Mechanical factors that prevent the expulsion of
rectal contents during increases in intra-abdominal pressure would block
defaecation unless prevented by an as yet unidentified compensatory mechanism. Moreover, since an increase in abdominal pressure will be transmitted to
the rectal contents, the pressures on either side of the rectal wall should be
equal and there should be no residual force to press the anterior rectal wall
down on the top of the anal canal. The latter can only occur if the ampulla recti
is empty and the anal pressure remains lower than the abdominal pressure.

We recently investigated the validity of the flap valve and flutter valve
mechanisms using a multi-lumen catheter to measure anal (three sites) and
rectal pressures in normal subjects and patients with faecal incontinence
during stepwise increases in intra-abdominal pressure. Our subjects were
instructed to blow into a tube connected to a sphygmomanometer, maintain-

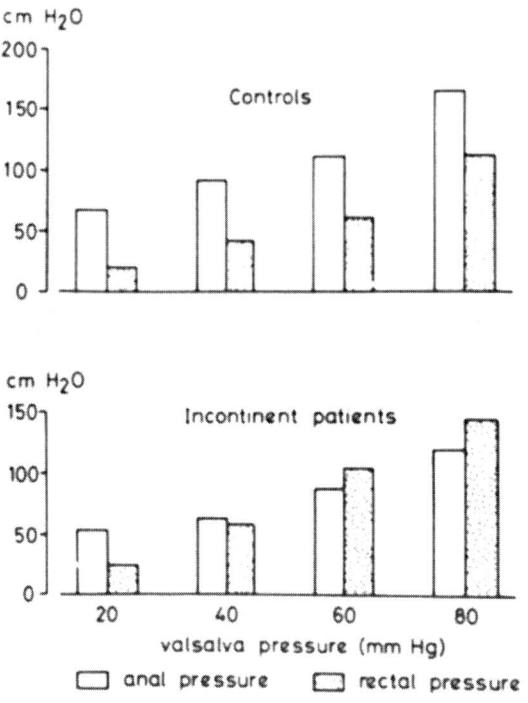

Figure 1. The relationship between the pressure in the rectum and the highest pressure in the anal canal in normal volunteers (top) and incontinent patients during stepwise increases in intra-abdominal pressures.

ing the level of mercury at prescribed levels using the diaphragm and abdominal muscles and not by apposing the tongue and palate.

For a flap valve to operate, the rectal pressure would have to be greater than the anal pressure as the intra-abdominal pressure rose. A flutter valve would require both anal and rectal pressures to increase by roughly equivalent amounts as the intra-abdominal pressure rose. Our results showed that neither of these situations exist in normal subjects; the anal pressure remained higher than the rectal pressure as subjects increased their intra-abdominal pressures (Figure 1). This situation could only be produced by a reflex increase in anal contractility caused by an increase in abdominal pressure, and perhaps initiated by stretch receptors on the pelvic floor [3]. Previous observations have shown that the external sphincter and puborectalis muscle increase their activity as subjects cough, talk and strain [4, 5], and there are strong correlations between the electrical activity in the striated muscles in the pelvic floor and both intra-abdominal pressure and anal pressure [6]. Thus the data suggest that during increases in intra-abdominal pressure, continence is normally preserved by a compensatory increase in the contraction of the striated muscles of the pelvic floor.

The conditions for the operation of a flap valve do exist, however, if the anal sphincter is abnormally weak. In patients with faecal incontinence, the anal pressure may fall below the rectal pressure as the intra-abdominal pressure rises (Figure 1) and if the rectum is empty the anterior rectal wall would be forced into the anal canal. If the rectum contains fluid, however, leakage takes place as the intra-abdominal pressure rises above the anal pressure. Thus, even though the conditions exist for a flap valve, this does not prevent incontinence when the rectum contains fluid. The failure of the anal pressures to keep ahead of the rises in intra-abdominal pressure in these patients can be explained either by weakness of the puborectalis and external sphincter or by an impaired sensory component of the reflex or both. Rises in intra-abdominal pressure are probably detected by stretch receptors in the levatores ani. Recent measurements of the electrical activity of the puborectalis and external anal sphincter indicate that larger intra-abdominal pressures are required to increase the activity of these muscles in incontinent patients compared with normal subjects [6], although the tonic activity of these muscles at rest may be quite normal. This 'deferred recruitment' of striated muscle would not only contribute to the incontinence, it would also explain the perineal descent seen in so many incontinent subjects [7], since rises in intra-abdominal pressure would cause the poorly responsive muscles to stretch further before they started to contract.

If the postulated flap valve does not contribute to faecal continence, is the acute angulation between the anus and rectum important? Patients with idiopathic faecal incontinence have a more obtuse ano-rectal angles than normal subjects [7] but this may be secondary to abnormal descent of the pelvic floor. Acute ano-rectal angulation would not affect continence to fluid unless the puborectalis sling was compressing the upper anal canal against a relatively immobile solid object. Perhaps the cervix uteri serves this function in the female and the prostate in the male, though there is no evidence to support either of these possibilities. The function of the ano-rectal angle in maintaining continence to solids is more clear since considerable rectal pressures would be required to mould a solid cylindrical stool around such an acute angle.

Responses to rectal distension

The challenge to the continence mechanism produced by rectal distension has been simulated by infusing 1500 ml of saline into the rectum at a rapid rate (60 ml/min^{-1}) [8]. Measurements of ano-rectal pressures and the electrical activity of the external anal sphincter (EAS) during this provocative test [9] can provide insights into the mechanisms by which continence is maintained in normal subjects and the events that cause leakage in incontinent patients.

136

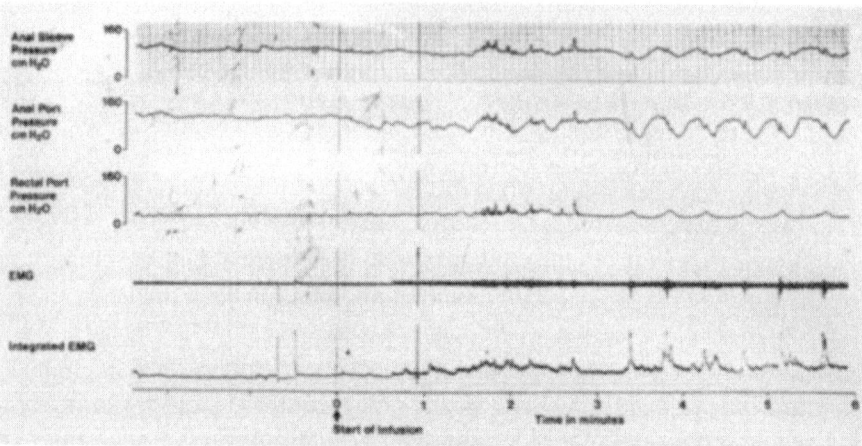

Figure 2. A recording of ano-rectal pressures and external anal sphincter EMG in a normal subject before and after the onset of rectal infusion of saline.

In normal subjects, rectal infusion of saline induces a regular series of events, consisting of rectal contractions, relaxations of the internal anal sphincter (IAS) and increases in external and sphincter (EAS) activity (Figure 2). These coordinated events occur at intervals of approximately one minute. A single coordinated event can be induced by rapid distension of a balloon in the rectum. On the basis of current knowledge it seems likely that stimulation of stretch receptors in the rectal wall (with saline or a balloon) causes a contraction of the rectum and a relaxation of the IAS through intrinsic reflexes that can be modulated by extrinsic nerves [10, 11]. Contraction of the striated muscles of the EAS and puborectalis in response to rectal distension is mediated by a spinal reflex [5] but probably requires conscious perception of rectal distension for its full expression.

Continence appears to be maintained during rectal infusion of saline by the residual tone of the sphincter during anal relaxation [9]. The brief phasic contraction of the EAS appeared to contribute little to continence during rectal infusion since it occurred before the deepest relaxation of the IAS and the rectal pressure peak which was in any case always lower than the anal pressure. It seems likely that contraction of the EAS makes the major contribution to the residual sphincter pressure, since IAS tone appears to be inhibited maximally during inflation of a rectal balloon with relatively small volumes (50 ml) of air, and the initial phasic response of the EAS to rectal distension is followed by an increased level of activity that remains above basal values for as long as the balloon remains inflated (Figure 3). Deflation of the balloon then evokes another brief burst before the activity in the EAS returns to basal values.

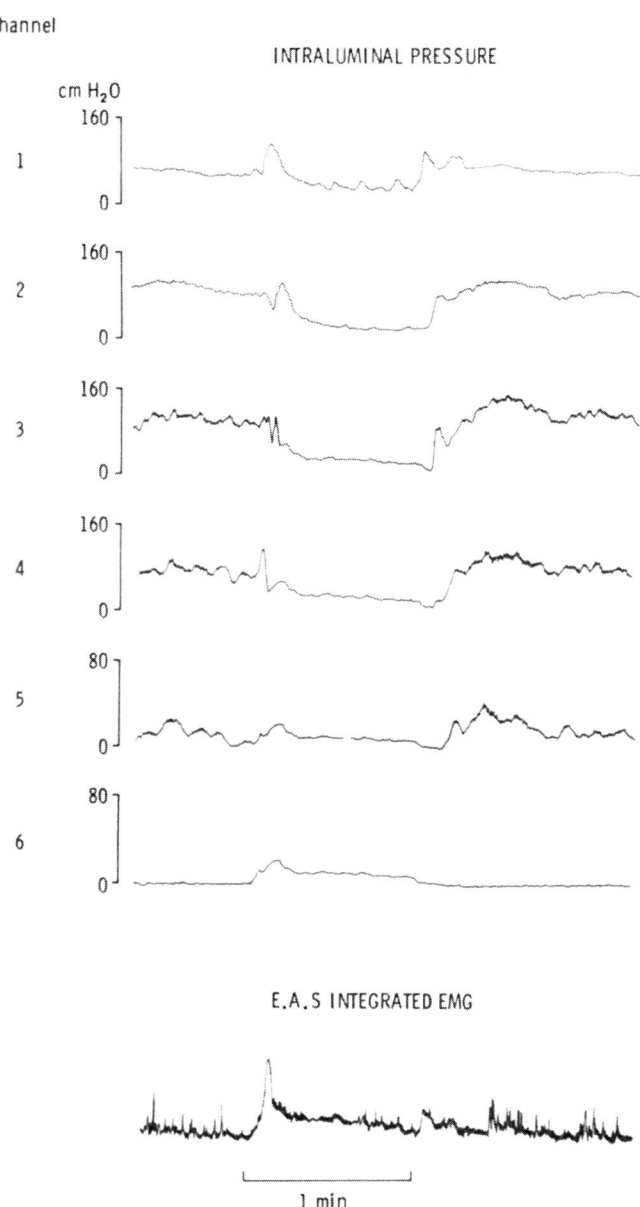

Figure 3. The effect of inflation of a rectal balloon with 50 ml air on the pressures recorded at six sites in the anal canal, each separated by 0.5 cm and on the external anal sphincter EMG. Note that the electrical activity in the EAS remains elevated as long as the balloon remains inflated.

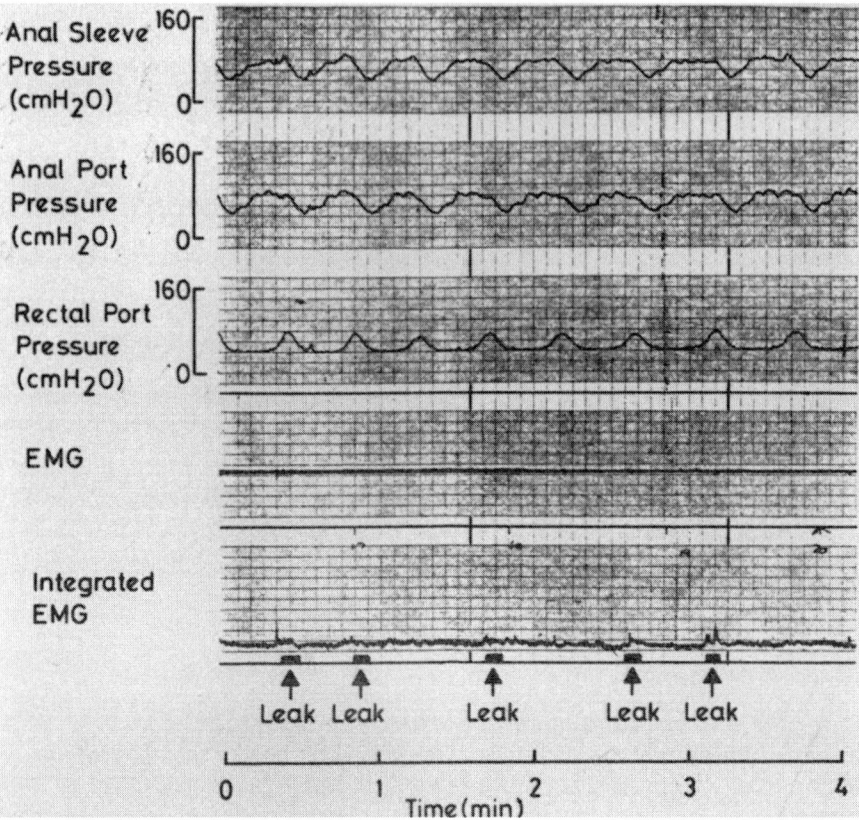

Figure 4. A typical record of anal and rectal pressure fluctuations and external sphincter EMG during rectal infusion of saline in an incontinent patient. Increases in rectal pressure are associated with anal relaxations and low-amplitude increases in external sphincter EMG. In this patient, external sphincter contractions do not appear on the anal sleeve channel.

Inadequate external sphincter response

Two distinct patterns of ano-rectal activity were seen in incontinent patients during rectal infusion of saline [12]. In some patients, saline infusion induced normal rectal contractions and IAS relaxations, but there was little or no compensatory activity in the EAS (Figure 4). Leakage of saline occurred during rectal contraction and IAS relaxation, when the rectal pressure equalled or exceeded the anal pressure. Incontinence in this group of patients appeared to be related to a defective external sphincter response to rectal distension.

External sphincter weakness and incontinence is particularly common in multiparous women. To explain this it has been suggested that the pelvic floor can be weakened during labour and subsequent straining at stool will cause gross perineal descent. The latter may occur partly because the stretch receptors that mediate pelvic floor contraction in response to increases in intra-abdominal pressure are desensitised. An abnormal degree of perineal descent is thought to stretch and compress the pudendal nerve as it winds around the ischial spine to enter the perineum, resulting after a few years in neuropathic weakness of the EAS [13, 14].

A defective external sphincter response to rectal distension may also be caused by diminished rectal or anal sensation. Normal people can detect distension of the rectum at levels lower than those which cause IAS relaxation, alerting them to the threat of incontinence and allowing them to prevent this by contracting the pelvic floor. Impaired sensory awareness of rectal distension has been found in incontinent patients with diabetes mellitus [15], meningomyelocele [16], faecal impaction in the elderly [15], children with encopresis [18] and in some patients with idiopathic faecal incontinence. Many of these patients are unable to perceive rectal distension at levels that cause internal sphincter relaxation, and in consequence may fail to contract their external sphincter to prevent incontinence. In some patients, sensory awareness of rectal distension may be delayed so that contraction of the EAS occurs too late to prevent incontinence as the sphincter relaxes [19]. Biofeedback training has been used to enhance EAS response to rectal distension in such patients [16, 20], while sensory retraining can facilitate the early detection of small rectal volumes. The situation is much worse in elderly patients with faecal impaction [17] and patients with low spinal lesions because anal and peri-anal sensations may be absent as well. Such patients may be unaware that they have been incontinent until they notice that their clothes are soiled.

Ano-rectal irritability

Incontinent patients, who show a normal pattern of internal sphincter relaxation in response to rectal infusion of saline also exhibit rectal pressures that are higher than normal [12]. Serial distension of a rectum of such patients with increasing volumes of air shows that the anus relaxes more profoundly at lower volumes than normal subjects (unpublished observations). These data suggest that these patients have a degree of rectal irritability and intolerance to lower rectal volumes, and resemble the published results from patients with the irritable bowel syndrome [21]. High rectal pressure and precipitous anal relaxation in response to rectal distension are particularly likely to cause incontinence if rectal sensation or external sphincter contraction is impaired.

The rectum may become more sensitive to rectal distension if the rectal contents are irritant. We have found that the incorporation of as little as 1 mM deoxycholic acid into the rectal infusion of saline increases rectal contractility

140

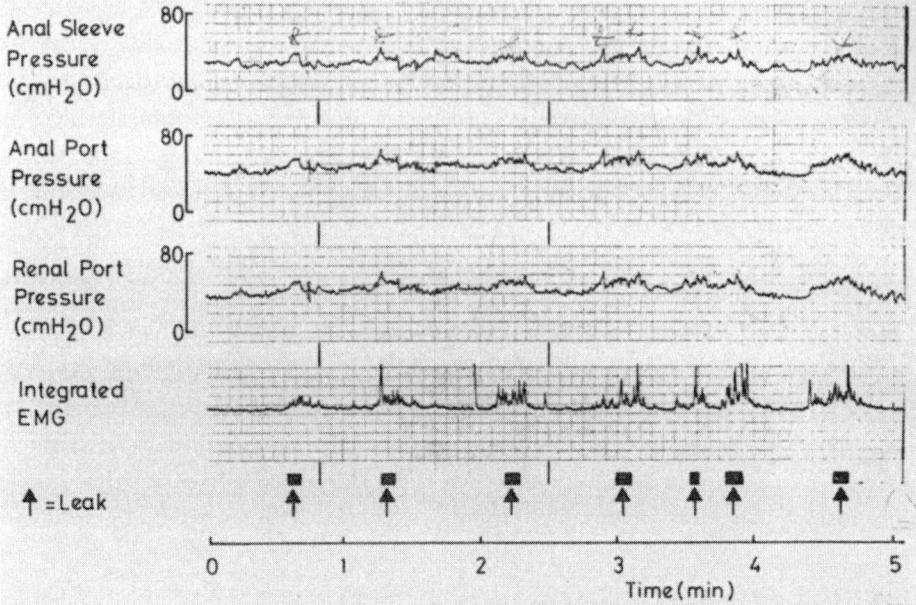

Figure 5. A typical record of anal and rectal pressure fluctuations and external sphincter electromyogram (EMG) during rectal infusion of saline in an incontinent patient. Identical pressure profiles are seen throughout the ano-rectum. These are associated with a similar profile in the integrated EMG.

and reduces the volume of fluid that could be infused into the rectum before leakage occurred (unpublished observations).

Impaired internal sphincter contraction

Recordings from 59% of the patients, studied by rectal infusion of saline, were characterised by clusters of irregular contractions, visible throughout the ano-rectum and similar in profile to the integrated record of the electrical activity of the EAS [12] (Figure 5). The resting anal tone in these patients was abnormally low [12], and showed a sustained reduction soon after the infusion commenced. Thus the IAS appeared weak and easily inhibited so that the record was dominated by the phasic increases in the activity of the EAS. In the absence of IAS contraction, the ano-rectum behaved like a common cavity squeezed by contractions of the EAS and puborectalis. Leakage occurs during these contractions, and may be explained by at least two possible mechanisms. Either rectal contractions force saline through the sphincter, the external sphincter contracting too late as the subject perceives fluid in the anal canal or in the peri-anal skin, or regular contractions of the puborectalis compress the fluid in the ano-rectal cavity forcing it through a weak external sphincter.

There are several possible mechanisms by which weakness of the internal anal sphincter will lead to incontinence if the external sphincter and puborectalis are contracting normally. The internal sphincter normally shields the sensory receptors in the mid-anal canal from rectal contents [22]. Relaxation of the IAS upon rectal distension exposes these receptors to rectal contents while activity in the external sphincter keeps the lower anal canal closed. This warns the subject of the imminence of incontinence and allows him to reinforce the contraction of the external sphincter. If the internal sphincter is abnormally weak, then the anal receptors could become desensitised by continuous exposure to rectal contents or the external sphincter could become fatigued by a constant stimulus to contract. An alternative explanation is that the internal sphincter may require mechanical support from the striated muscles of the pelvic floor in order to contract effectively. The abnormally low maximum squeeze pressures observed in these patients and the marked pelvic floor descent [6, 7] leads us to speculate that the weak puborectalis and EAS permits the traction of the stretched levatores ani to oppose the intrinsic contraction of the IAS.

Spontaneous relaxation

We have recently observed that the anal pressure in some incontinent patients can exhibit periods of profound and prolonged relaxation that are not associated with rectal distension. The basal anal pressures and the pressures recorded during a maximum squeeze in these patients are not necessarily abnormally low, although upon spontaneous relaxation, anal pressures may drop to zero. The reason for this phenomenon is unknown, though transient and shallow relaxations occur in normal subjects in association with contractions that are recorded throughout the rectum.

The role of the anal cushions

Minor degrees of seepage are common after haemorrhoidectomy and a few patients may be considerably distressed by frank incontinence after this operation. In a recent study, we measured the anal pressures in response to probes of increasing diameters. From these data we calculated the wall tension and we observed that at zero tension, when the circular muscle fibres are as short as possible, the canal would have a finite diameter; in other words the data suggested that the muscles surrounding the anal canal would be unable to close the aperture unless assisted in some way by the mucosal lining. The anal cushions have been compared to erectile tissue with large blood spaces and

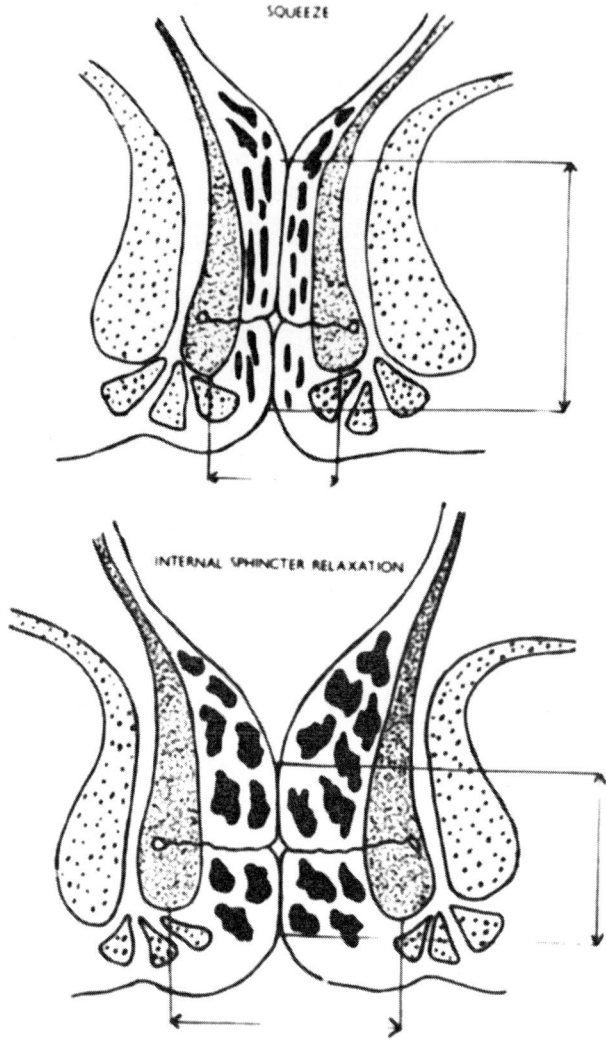

Figure 6. A diagram illustrating the expansion of the anal cushions to fill the anal canal as the anal sphincter relaxes.

direct arteriovenous connections [23] (Figure 6). Thus the pressure in these structures lies probably somewhere between arterial and venous pressures. If this were the case, then the vascular pressure in the anal cushions would contribute to the anal pressure, while the distension of the anal canal by the turgor of the cushions would stretch the concentric muscle fibres and allow them to contract with greater efficiency. The anal cushions could also be compressed to allow the passage of a stool but swell to close off the anal canal under resting conditions. Similar erectile tissue exists around the urethral sphincter.

Conclusions

In conclusion, we would propose that most cases of faecal incontinence are caused by abnormalities in the response of the EAS and puborectalis to rectal distension/contraction or to increases in intra-abdominal pressure. Such abnormalities may affect the afferent or the efferent limb of these responses. Mechanical factors, such as the flap valve, are not responsible for the maintenance of continence in normal subjects, but could, in theory, help to preserve continence in patients who have abnormal weakness of the anal canal. On theoretical grounds, it appears that the anal cushions may help to preserve continence by acting as expansile balloons to seal the anal aperture and to permit the concentric muscle fibres to operate at optimum efficiency.

References

1. Parks AG, Porter NW, Hardcastle JD. 1966. The syndrome of the descending perineum. Proc R Soc Med 59: 477–482.
2. Phillips SF, Edwards DAW. 1965. Some aspects of anal continence and defaecation. Gut 6: 396–405.
3. Winkler G. 1958. Remarques sur la morphologie et l'innervation du muscle releveur de l'anus. Archives Anatomie et Histologie et Embryologie, Strasbourg 41: 77–95.
4. Floyd WF, Walls EW. 1953. Electromyography of the sphincter ani externus in man. J. Physiol 122: 599–609.
5. Parks AG, Porter NW, Melzack J. 1962. Experimental study of the reflex mechanism controlling the muscles of the pelvic floor. Dis Colon Rectum 5: 407–414.
6. Womack NR, Morrison JFB, Williams NS. 1986. Sensory impairment and muscle weakness combine to cause an inadequate anal sphincter in idiopathic faecal incontinence (IFI). Gut 27: A624–A625.
7. Bartolo DDC, Read NW, Jarratt JA, Read MG, Donnelly TC, Johnson AG. 1983. Differences in anal sphincter function and clinical presentation in patients with pelvic floor descent. Gastroenterology 85: 68–75.
8. Read NW, Harford WV, Schmulen AC, Read MG, Santa-Ana C, Fordtran JS. 1979. A clinical study of patients with faecal incontinence and diarrhoea. Gastroenterology 76: 747–756.
9. Haynes WG, Read NW. 1982. Ano-rectal activity in man during rectal infusion of saline: a dynamic assessment of the anal continence mechanism. J Physiol 330: 45–56.
10. White JC, Verlot MG, Ehrentheil O. 1940. Neurogenic disturbances of the colon and their investigation by the colonmetrogram. Annals of Surgery 112: 1042–1057.
11. Meunier P, Mollard P. 1977. Control of the internal anal sphincter (manometric study with human subjects). Pflugers Arch für die gesamte Physiologie des Menschen unter der Tiere. 370: 233–239.

144

12. Read NW, Haynes WG, Bartolo DCC, Hall J, Read MG, Donnelly TC, Johnson AG. 1983. Use of ano-rectal manometry during rectal infusion of saline to investigate sphincter function in incontinent patients. Gastroenterology 85: 105–113.
13. Snooks SJ, Henry MM, Swash M. 1985. Ano-rectal incontinence and rectal prolapse: differential assessment of the innervation to puborectalis and external anal sphincter muscles. Gut 26: 470–476.
14. Parks AG, Swash M, Urich H. 1977. Sphincter denervation in ano-rectal incontinence and rectal prolapse. Gut 18: 656–665.
15. Wald A, Tunnguntla AK. 1984. Ano-rectal sensation dysfunction in faecal incontinence and diabetes mellitus. N Engl J Med 310: 1282–1287.
16. Wald A. 1983. Biofeedback for neurogenic faecal incontinence: rectal sensation is a determinant of outcome. J Paed Gastroenterology and Nutrition 2: 302–306.
17. Read NW, Abouzekry L. 1986. Why do patients with faecal impaction have faecal incontinence? Gut 27: 283–287.
18. Molnar D, Taitz LS, Urwin OM, Wales JKM. 1983. Ano-rectal manometry results in defaecation disorders. Arch Dis Childhood 58: 257–261.
19. Buser WD, Miner PB. 1985. Successful treatment of delayed rectal sensation with related faecal incontinence by ano-rectal manometry. Gastroenterology 88: A1339.
20. Cerulli MA, Nikoomanesh P, Schuster MM. 1979. Progress of biofeedback conditioning for faecal incontinence. Gastroenterology 76: 742–746.
21. Schuster MM. 1985. Ano-rectal disorder in the irritable bowel syndrome. In: Read NW (ed.) Irritable Bowel Syndrome. Grune & Stratton, London, pp. 191–202.
22. Bennett RC, Duthie HL. 1964. The functional importance of the internal sphincter. Br J Surg 51: 355–357.
23. Thompson WMF. 1975. The nature of haemorrhoids. Br J Surg 62: 542–552.

3.5 Medical treatment

Ph.B. MINER, Jr.

Introduction

The treatment goal for patients with faecal incontinence is to eliminate or decrease the number of involuntary passages of faeces. Numerous causes for the symptom of faecal incontinence are recognised suggesting successful treatment approaches will vary. Medical management is limited since few drugs have been shown to alter the symptoms or the observable abnormalities in patients with faecal incontinence. It seems unlikely that medical treatment can be effective for patients with irreversible muscle and nerve damage, which has been reported to be present in as high as 80% of the cases of faecal incontinence [1]. Rational treatment is limited further by the imprecise understanding of the complex process of voluntary defaecation and continence. Until proper studies provide sufficient information to direct drugs at specific and treatable abnormalities, medical management will consist of partial treatment of some of the factors involved in the continence mechanism or in designing a program of planned defaecation to avoid incontinent episodes.

Current drugs available for treatment of faecal incontinence

Medical treatment of faecal incontinence begins with appropriate management of any underlying disease which may contribute to gastro-intestinal symptoms. For example, faecal incontinence related to ulcerative colitis often responds to the successful treatment of the inflamed colonic mucosa with steroids and sulfasalazine. Unless a specific, treatable disease has been overlooked, this suggestion is not very helpful.

The wide range of diseases associated with faecal incontinence makes grouping of patients by manometric findings a better clinical classification. The author in a recent study of 29 patients with faecal incontinence due to a number of different problems divided patients into three principle groups on the basis of resting and squeeze anal canal pressures, the volume of rectally infused saline patients were able to retain, and the volume of their diarrhoea [2]. The largest proportion of patients (60%) had low anal sphincter pressures, a low stool volume and incontinence to rectally infused saline. Drugs which could enhance resting and/or squeeze anal sphicter pressures may be helpful for these patients. Patients with the second pattern (30%) had normal anal canal pressures and stool volumes, but incontinence to saline infused rectally. The faecal incontinence in these cases does not appear amenable to pharmacologic manipulation. The smallest group (10%) had normal anal canal pressures and high stool volumes. Decreasing stool volume should improve faecal incontinence in this small group of patients. Loperamide [3, 4], lomotil [4, 5] and codeine [4] delay the passage of bowel contents in the colon allowing a greater percentage of the stool water to be absorbed. Palmer et al. [4] evaluated the effect of loperamide, lomotil and codeine on the frequency of stools in patients with chronic diarrhoea. There was a decrease in the number of stools per day and greater number of solid stools in their patients. They suggest these drugs accounted for the observed improvement in faecal incontinence. Harford et al. [5] examined the effect of diphenoxylate on ano-rectal function in patients with diarrhoea and faecal incontinence. No changes were found in anal canal basal and squeeze pressures nor in the saline continence test allowing them to conclude the symptomatic improvement was due to the reduction in stool weight and stool frequency. Unfortunately, faecal incontinence in this study was poorly documented and no patients had incontinence during any phase of the study. Of these drugs, loperamide is the only drug which has been successfully shown to improve faecal incontinence in a placebo controlled study directed at the control of faecal incontinence [3]. Loperamide (12 mg per day) reduced the number of episodes of urgency and incontinence while stool consistency improved and stool weight was reduced. Internal anal sphincter (IAS) pressure increased and patients were able to retain a larger volume of rectally infused saline. The ability of an individual to retain 1500 ml of saline tests the voluntary strength of the sphincteric barrier against the physical stress of fluid in the rectum and the pressure generated by colonic and rectal contractions against the sphincter. The amount of saline infused prior to the first leak appears to be one of the best predictors of faecal incontinence [2, 6]. Although the change in the character of the stool after loperamide [3] undoubtedly contributed to the decrease in the number of incontinent stools, the enhanced saline retention suggests the increased IAS pressure plays an important role in the successful treatment of these patients. Since patients with IAS weakness are at high risk for liquid stool incontinence [7], loperamide may improve continence in these patients by increasing IAS pressure and firming stool consistency. Based on the categorisation of patients by ano-rectal function, loperamide appears superior to codeine and dephenoxylate in the group of patients with low sphincter pressures although the drugs seem similar with regard to the ability to decrease stool volume.

Potential role of bile acid binding resins in faecal incontinence

Bile acid malabsorption causes diarrhoea by inducing colonic secretion of water and stimulating the motility of the sigmoid colon [8]. The proposal that bile salt malabsorption causes faecal incontinence in patients is complicated by the presence of underlying diseases such as Crohn's disease, radiation proctitis and peptic ulcer disease after vagotomy in patients known to have bile salt malabsorption. Thaysen and Pedersen have described three carefully evaluated patients with chronic diarrhoea due to idiopathic bile salt malabsorption [9]. In this clinical description of idiopathic bile salt catharsis, one patient clearly had faecal incontinence as a major symptom prior to treatment and another appears to have had faecal incontinence as implied by the discussion of her course after cholestyramine treatment. The clinical improvement in all of the patients symptoms after cholestyramine treatment provides important support for the hypothesis that bile acid malabsorption contributes to faecal incontinence and bile acid binding resins are useful in management of the diarrhoea and incontinence.

There is considerable evidence in experimental animals that bile acids stimulate colonic motility. Flynn et al. summarised these studies and evaluated the effect of 5–25mM concentrations of cholate, chenodeoxycholate and deoxycholate on colonic myoelectrical activity in dogs with Thiry-Vella loops [10]. Cholic acid and chenodeoxycholic acid did not change motility at any of the concentrations tested while a 15mM deoxycholic acid perfusion markedly increased the motility index in the loops. This increased activity was inhibited by cholestyramine. Bannister and Read (personal communication) have conducted preliminary experiments on the effect of rectal bile acid infusion in normal volunteers. After 500 ml of a 3mM deoxycholic acid solution infused into the rectum, the volunteers became more sensitive to balloon distension with a lower balloon volumes inducing a strong desire to defaecate. The stimulation was sufficiently strong in half the volunteers that they were unable to retain the fluid long enough to have the tests completed. Further testing is needed to understand the reason for the rectal sensitivity to bile acids, but the effect on these simple ano-rectal tests suggests a potentially important role for bile salts in patients with ano-rectal dysfunction. In the sigmoid colon, similar experiments in normal volunteers were performed by Taylor et al. [8]. They perfused the sigmoid colon with cholic, chenodeoxycholic and deoxycholic acid in 5mM concentrations. Rectal pressures were recorded with an open-tip tube and were not altered by bile salt infusion. Electrical activity, recorded from the rectal wall by monopolar suction electrode, was significantly increased after the infusion of 15mM deoxycholic acid. These studies suggest bile salt malabsorption stresses the continence mechanism by increasing colonic fluid secretion, altering perception of rectal contents and increasing colorectal motor activity.

With the exception of idiopathic bile salt catharsis, the clinical importance of bile salts in the management of faecal incontinence is speculative and not supported by good scientific evidence. Many gastroenterologists have found cholestyramine useful in selected patients with incontinence despite the lack of good scientific data. Crohn's disease is the most easily recognised clinical problem with bile acid malabsorption. The complex pathology in patients with Crohn's disease weakens the argument in favour of faecal incontinence induced by bile acids. In a study of urgency in Crohn's disease [11], all patients with urgency (9 of 20 had incontinence) had small bowel involvement and many had no evidence of large bowel, rectal, or perineal disease. No important changes were present in either basal or squeeze pressures in the anal canal in the patients with or without urgency. The absence of disease in the colon and rectum in many patients, supports the speculation that an increased bowel fluid or stimulated colonic motility may be involved in the urgency and incontinence in Crohn's disease. The required presence of disease in the terminal ileum makes bile acid induced changes highly likely. Cholestyramine treatment should decrease urgency and incontinence in some patients with Crohn's disease by improving stool consistency and limiting active colonic motility induced by bile acids.

It is not generally appreciated that bile acid malabsorption is a common sequela of pelvic irradiation. The terminal ileum is often involved in the radiation field due to its low position in the pelvis. The obvious mucosal changes in the colon visible after irradiation are believed to be responsible for the diarrhoea while the poor fluid absorption and decreased rectal compliance may be responsible for faecal incontinence. Ludgate and Merrick examined 26 patients with post-pelvic irradiation induced diarrhoea by using a radio-labelled bile acid conjugate and B_{12} [12]. Incontinence is not mentioned in this paper. Fifty percent of the patients malabsorbed the bile acid alone and 12/13 responded to cholestyramine. A further 11% had abnormal absorption of both isotopes and responded to treatment with cholestyramine. This excellent response rate indicates the importance of bile acids in this clinical disorder and offers a good therapeutic choice for patients with post-irradiation diarrhoea and faecal incontinence.

Patients with irritable bowel syndrome (IBS) are the most interesting subset of patients in whom bile acid malabsorption may be important. Patients with IBS are present in most studies on faecal incontinence. Often they have normal or elevated anal canal pressures. Taylor et al. in the study alluded to earlier [8] found perfusion of 5mM deoxycholic acid into the sigmoid colon of patients with irritable bowel syndrome produces a significant increase in the colonic motility. The colonic stimulation with concentrations below 15mM deoxycholic acid indicates greater sensitivity to bile acids in IBS patients than in normal volunteers. Merrick et al. found 5 of 42 patients with irritable bowel syndrome had bile acid malabsorption by the SeHCAT [13] strengthening the plausibility of the association. Proposing bile acid malabsorption may not be necessary as Taylor et al. found the level of bile salts in the faeces of patients with irritable bowel syndrome is sufficient to cause increased sigmoid motility.

The difficulty of management of these three groups of patients with faecal incontinence by conventional means warrants a judicious trial of cholestyramine in patients with faecal incontinence and Crohn's disease, radiation induced diarrhoea and irritable bowel syndrome. Proper prospective, blinded therapeutic trials may verify the use of cholestyramine and may provide additional information with regard to the importance of bile acids in faecal incontinence.

Role of training in control of faecal incontinence

Training programs are an important aspect of the medical management of faecal incontinence. They are designed to regain normal function or to plan defaecation to avoid incontinence. Biofeedback is the most successful training method improving about 70% of all patients with faecal incontinence [14]. Our approach to biofeedback has emphasised enhanced sensory perception of very low volumes of rectal balloon distension (less than 5 ml) in conjunction with shortening the time from balloon distension to sensory perception. Most of the patients in our current study have fewer incontinent episodes after sensory training alone. Further improvement occurs when muscle contraction is coordinated with balloon distension in the rectum permitting the patient to have a timely and maximal response to low volume stimulation. This method of faecal continence training emphasises the early recognition of a desire to defaecate and improved control of the muscles of the pelvic floor. Success in the use of biofeedback for patients with faecal incontinence makes this method the first step in patient management. A detailed discussion of the success of biofeedback is presented in another section of this book.

'Planned defaecation' is an important though often overlooked method of managing the problem of faecal incontinence. Most patients have already tried to determine when they will be incontinent so they may adjust their daily pattern of activities. Bulk laxatives provide stools of predictable size and consistency while making bowel actions more regular. In selected patients this approach may suffice. Glycerin suppositories used in the morning stimulate bowel evacuation when the patient can control his access to a toilet and permit him to be free of soiling for the rest of the day. This approach to the management of faecal incontinence may be very successful in the elderly patient with poor recognition of rectal fullness or in children with incontinence associated with constipation.

Planned defaecation is convenient in many patients with faecal incontinence but mandatory in most patients with spinal injuries [15], although a select number of patients improve after biofeedback. Wald has been able to train some patients with limited disability due to meningomyelocele and sensory thresholds below 20 ml balloon distension [16]. A few spinal injury patients may require or desire a colostomy to allow them control of the incontinence but the vast majority manage by using a planned bowel evacuation program. Spinal cord injury patients can be divided into two principle groups based on the presence of the reflexes mediated through the spinal cord. In patients with sacral lesions, the internal anal sphincter pressure is present but often low and rectal contractions are markedly decreased making evacuation difficult. A few patients have incomplete disruption of the parasympathetics and automatic defaecation may occur after digital stimulation of the anal sphincter and puborectalis. In suprasacral lesions, the IAS has normal resting tone and responds to rectal distension by relaxation. Although the relaxation is mediated through the intramural nerves, it is useful in allowing automatic defaecation. Since pressure and the tone in the sigmoid colon and the rectum are intact, process of defaecation proceeds normally once it has been stimulated by pressure on the anal sphincter and puborectalis. Spinal lesions which can be managed using automatic defaecation can be predicted by EAS contraction to pinprick stimulation within one cm of the anus ('anal wink').

Suprasacral lesions must be further divided into two broad categories – quadraplegics and paraplegics. In both groups, medical management consists of planned colonic evacuation every other day and dietary restriction to limit episodes of loose stools. Quadraplegics often find planned defaecation is easiest while they are in bed. The loss of motor function of the trunk makes it difficult, if not impossible for quadraplegics to balance on the toilet for the time necessary to evacuate the bowels. The second problem with lesions above the sympathetic ganglion (Th-5) is autonomic dysfunction which accompanies defaecation. While the patient is attempting to pass the bowel motion, the blood pressure rises, immediately falling after defaecation, to pressures low enough to cause syncope in an upright individual. Quadraplegics frequently require assistance due to the degree of their disability. The patient is positioned in a semi-recumbent position with a disposable sheet placed under him. The rectum is checked for stool and the puborectalis is stimulated with the examining finger. If defaecation is not routinely initiated by this examination, 2 ml of bisacodyl liquid or a microlax enema is gently introduced into the rectum. The use of the liquid is preferable to the alternative stimulating suppository since it has a rapid onset of action and there appears to be less of a chance of an 'echo' bowel motion several hours later. Non-stimulant glycerin suppositories may be used in place of the initial digital stimulation if they reliably initiate a bowel movement. After the bowel motion is completed, manual examination is done to check and empty the rectum if necessary. The patient should be able to remain unsoiled for the next one to two days. Paraplegics follow a similar training regimen, although they are more independent as they can transfer to the toilet and sit upright without assistance. In many patients with suprasacral lesions, stimulation every other day is sufficient to prevent soiling.

Patients with sacral lesions are more difficult to manage, since they have not only sphincter weakness, but impaired emptying of the sigmoid colon and rectum. Stool softeners should be used to prevent the occurrence of hard stools, which may damage the anal canal when passed. Bulk laxatives are occasionally helpful, but often produce a large, soft and unmanageable bowel motion. Digital stimulation can occasionally be successful, but most often, manual evacuation is needed to clear the rectum on a regular (often twice a day) basis.

Future drug development

Theoretically, there are several drugs which can manipulate the measurable abnormalities of the ano-rectum. One of our recently studied patients with spontaneous and profound relaxation of the IAS provides an excellent example. He had periods of unrecognised anal canal relaxation lasting as long as 120 seconds with a decrease in basal pressure to ten percent of the resting pressure. His principal symptom was frequent diarrhoea with marked urgency and faecal incontinence. He had many systemic symptoms suggestive of systemic mastocytosis including, debilitating headaches, flushing, pruritis, acid peptic symptoms and fatigue. A skin biopsy revealed an excessive number of mast cells. Since histamine release causes many of the symptoms in this disorder, a trial of histamine blockers was given. This treatment diminished the systemic symptoms and caused the basal anal canal pressure to increase from 120 to 160 mm H_2O and modified the spontaneous anal sphincter relaxations. Although histamine is known to cause the IAS to relax [17], this is the first instance in which histamine receptor blockers have been shown to increase basal anal sphincter tone.

Histamine antagonists, anticholinergic drugs, adrenergic agonists and prostaglandin synthesis inhibitors need to be evaluated for their effects on anorectal physiology and their possible contribution to the management of the difficult clinical problem of faecal incontinence.

152

References

1. Swash M. 1985. New concepts in incontinence. Br Med J 290: 4–5.
2. Read NW, Harford WV, Schmulen AC, Read MG, Santa-Ana C, Fordtran JS. 1979. A clinical study of patients with faecal incontinence and diarrhoea. Gastroenterology 76: 745–756.
3. Read MG, Read NW, Barber DC, Duthie HL. 1982. Effects of loperamide on anal sphincter function in patients complaining of chronic diarrhoea with faecal incontinence and urgency. Dig Dis Sci 27: 807–813.
4. Palmer KR, Corbett CL, Holdsworth CD. 1980. Double-blind cross-over study comparing loperamide, codeine and diphenoxylate in the treatment of chronic diarrhoea. Gastroenterology 79: 1272–1275.
5. Harford WV, Krejs GJ, Santa-Ana CA, Fordtran JS. 1980. Acute effect of diphenoxylate with atropine (Lomotil) in patients with chronic diarrhoea and faecal incontinence. Gastroenterology 78: 440–443.
6. Read NW, Haynes WG, Bartolo DCC, Hall J, Read MG, Donnelly TC, Johnson AG. 1983. Use of ano-rectal manometry during rectal infusion of saline to investigate sphincter function in incontinent patients. Gastroenterology 85: 105–113.
7. Read NW, Bartolo DCC, Read MG. 1984. Differences in anal function in patients with incontinence to solids and in patients with incontinence to liquids. Br J Surg 71: 39–42.
8. Taylor I, Basu P, Hammond P, Darby C, Flynn M. 1980. Effect of bile acid perfusion on colonic motor function in patients with the irritable bowel syndrome. Gut 21: 843–847.
9. Thaysen EH, Pedersen L. 1976. Idiopathic bile salt catharsis. Gut 17: 965–970.
10. Flynn M, Darby C, Hyland J, Hammond P, Taylor I. 1979. The effect of bile acids on colonic myoelectric activity. Br J Surg 66: 776–779.
11. Buchmann P, Kolb E, Alexander-Williams J. 1981. Pathogenesis of urgency in defaecation in Crohn's disease. Digestion 22: 310–316.
12. Ludgate SM, Merrick MV. 1985. The pathogenesis of post-irradiation chronic diarrhoea: management of SeHCAT and B_{12} absorption for differential diagnosis determines treatment. Clin Radiol 36: 275–278.
13. Merrick MV, Eastwood MA, Ford MJ. 1985. Is bile acid malabsorption underdiagnosed? An evaluation of accuracy of diagnosis by measurement of SeHCAT retention. Br Med J 290: 665–668.
14. Wald A. 1981. Biofeedback therapy for faecal incontinence. Ann Int Med 95: 146–149.
15. Guttmann L. 1976. Spinal Cord Injuries – Comprehensive Management and Research. Second Edition. Oxford. Blackwell Scientific Publications.
16. Wald A. 1983. Biofeedback for neurogenic faecal incontinence: rectal sensation is a determinant of outcome. J Pediatr Gastroenterol Nutr 2: 302–306.
17. Burleigh DE, D'Mello A, Parks AG. 1979. Responses of isolated human internal anal sphincter to drugs and electrical field stimulation. Gastroenterology 77: 484–490.

3.6 Biofeedback training and behavioural treatment

G. COREMANS & G. VANTRAPPEN

Introduction

Faecal incontinence is a disorder associated with considerable social and psychological repercussions. It may occur at all ages as the result of a large number of medical and surgical diseases impairing rectal sensation or affecting anal sphincter muscles or their nerve supply. It is particularly common in children and elderly patients. A multitude of therapies including bowel habit training programs, various types of sphincter repair, diets, drugs, and intra-anal plug electrodes yielded imperfect results. Biofeedback training seems to be a simple and efficient alternative to these treatment modalities and is likely to become an important tool in the management of conditions where there are problems of faecal incontinence. The method proved applicable to patients widely varying in age, severity of symptoms and in origin of their incontinence. Interestingly, biofeedback training that was promoted by the Johns Hopkins investigators for faecal incontinence derives its rationale and its methodology from the concepts of behavioural science [1, 2].

Biofeedback

Miller defined biofeedback as the use of modern instrumentation to give a person better moment-to-moment information about a specific physiologic process that is under control of the nervous system, but not clearly or accurately perceived [3]. In terms of servo systems this moment-to-moment information has been called feedback. In biologic feedback situations the physiological response is most of the time difficult to perceive, requiring mechanical or electronic equipment to register the response and to make it perceivable to the person who is learning. The type of learning involved in biofeedback training is not unique as it uses the same trial-and-error approach by which most motor skills are acquired. The subject learns from success or failure of

154

each attempt how to modify his performance to become more frequently successful [4].

Biofeedback is the basic component of operant conditioning as it is the basic component of all operant learning. The technique of operant conditioning simply reinforces a weak physiologic response by using biofeedback. A reward is given to reinforce the preceding weak response of a somatically or autonomically innervated structure. Information that the response is succeeding serves as a reward, and information that it is failing as a punishment [5].

Requirements for successful application of biofeedback

In general, operant conditioning can only be used for functional disorders in which a physiologic reaction can be monitored that is useful for feedback. To be useful in medicine feedback must be specific, i.e., the response that is used as feedback must represent a major symptom. Only the application of specific feedback is successful in generalising the response from the clinic to every day life [6].

Biofeedback not only must be specific, its display must also be sensitive, accurate and immediate [4]. The instrumentation must allow to register even small changes in the response. To avoid confusing the patient, the display should not report movement artefacts. A significant delay between the occurrence of a response and the perception of its occurrence will seriously impair the process of learning. A good feedback situation is having the subject watch a polygraph tracing as the physiologic process is monitored. Generalisation of the adequate (learned) response from the clinic to everyday life requires bidirectional training by alternating suppression and reinforcement of the response and by training with interpolated no-feedback trials [6].

In addition to these basic requirements for successful application of feedback there are certain characteristics of the subject that are important for the success of the feedback training. The individual must be motivated to learn and be able to understand and comply with the instructions [7]. Finally the trainer has to be convinced that only with patience can control of the impaired function be obtained.

Medical application of biofeedback

Biofeedback training resulted in significant lasting effects in the treatment of neuromuscular disorders, cardiac arrhythmias, postural hypotension and essential hypertension. Most successful, however, has been the use of feedback in the treatment of different types of faecal incontinence [2, 4, 6].

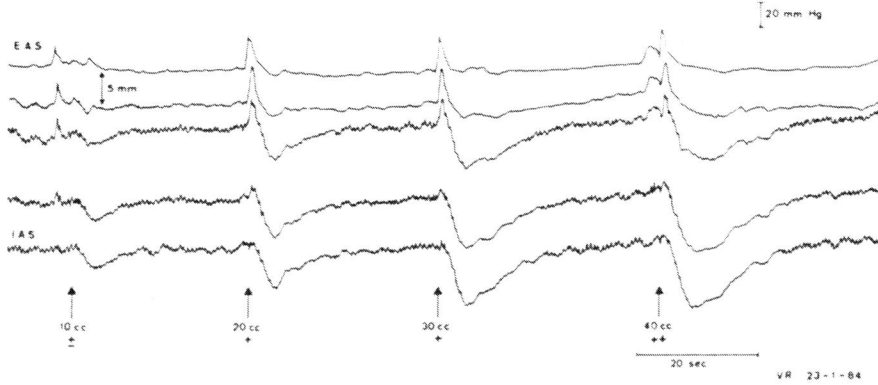

Figure 1. Rectosphincteric response in a normal subject recorded by a perfused catheter system. Rectal distension with increasing volumes of air induce reflex relaxations of the internal anal sphincter (IAS) and synchronous contractions of the external anal sphincter (EAS). The conscious sensitivity threshold is 20 cc.

Physiology and pathophysiology of faecal continence

In a normal subject, distension of a balloon within the rectum, which mimics the arrival of stool in this area, induces a reflex relaxation of the internal anal sphincter and a synchronous contraction of the external anal sphincter (Figure 1). The internal anal sphincter response is a true reflex, as internal anal sphincter inhibition is reliably elicited by rectal distension. The external sphincter contraction, on the other hand, seems to be a voluntary response rather than a reflex [9]. However, the external sphincter contraction is so habitual a response to rectal distension that it occurs automatically without conscious attention.

In the patient with faecal incontinence rectal distension induces normal relaxations of the internal sphincter, but no simultaneous contractions of the external sphincter (Figure 2). This situation where the arrival of stool in the rectum is followed by relaxation of the internal sphincter not accompanied by contraction of the voluntary sphincter, clearly predisposes to faecal incontinence. Because external anal sphincter response is initiated by the perception of rectal distension, faecal incontinence may arise in subjects who do not feel weak rectal distension or in whom the impaired sphincter can not prevent leakage of faecal matter [4]. The simultaneous contraction of the external sphincter which is cued by the perception of rectal distension is vital for the preservation of continence.

156

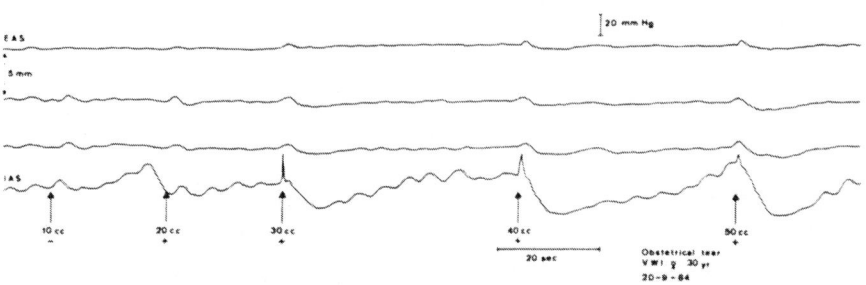

Figure 2. Rectosphincteric response in a patient (V.W.I.) with faecal incontinence secondary to fistulectomy before biofeedback training. Rectal distension with increasing volumes of air induce reflex relaxations of the internal anal sphincter (IAS). These relaxations are not accompanied by contractions of the external anal sphincter. The conscious sensitivity threshold is within normal range (20 cc).

Biofeedback situation in faecal incontinence

Biofeedback is classically provided by showing the patient the recording of anal sphincter pressures as they are being traced out by a polygraph. The pressures are recorded by two separate balloons or by a perfused catheter system, inserted into the anal canal. In the latter system the distance between the recording sites is 5 mm. The higher balloon or perfusion hole is partially surrounded by the internal anal sphincter, while the lower balloon or perfusion hole is partially surrounded by the external anal sphincter. Changes in tone of each sphincter muscle are transmitted via small waterfilled catheters to pressure transducers and displayed on a polygraph [4]. The electrical activity of the external anal sphincter can also be recorded by intra-anal ringelectrodes adapted to an electromyometer providing auditive feedback [10]. A larger balloon is located intra-rectally for transient distension of the rectum.

In patients with sphincteric faecal incontinence the major symptom, involuntary loss of faecal matter, correlates well with the registered physiologic response, i.e., the lowered pressure at the level of the anal sphincter. During the training the subject is asked to contract the external sphincter each time he senses distension (Figure 3).

Goals of biofeedback training

The most commonly employed biofeedback procedure includes three separate components, i.e., strengthening of voluntary sphincter muscle contraction,

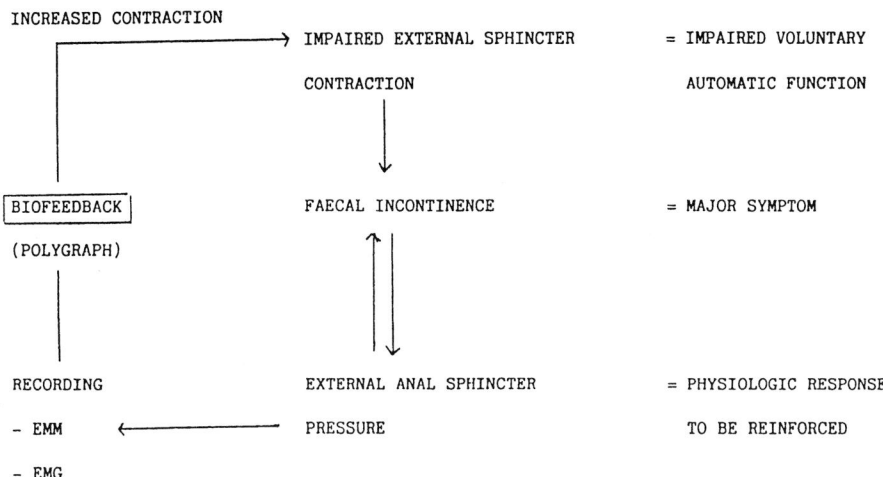

INCREASED CONTRACTION

IMPAIRED EXTERNAL SPHINCTER   = IMPAIRED VOLUNTARY

CONTRACTION   AUTOMATIC FUNCTION

BIOFEEDBACK   FAECAL INCONTINENCE   = MAJOR SYMPTOM

(POLYGRAPH)

RECORDING   EXTERNAL ANAL SPHINCTER   = PHYSIOLOGIC RESPONSE

- EMM   PRESSURE   TO BE REINFORCED

- EMG

Figure 3. The biofeedback situation in detail.

training in discrimination of the rectal sensation and training in synchronising the internal and external sphincter responses to distension [1]. The patients are taught to strengthen the sphincter muscle by allowing them to see or to hear the results of their efforts during maximal voluntary contraction (Figure 4). Instant auditory or visual feedback is provided by the already described instrumentation. The patient is encouraged to try to increase his response to make it appear more normal. In patients with lesions involving the afferent nerve pathways resulting in loss of rectal sensation, a threshold decrease can be obtained by conditioning them by gradually decreasing the distending volume. In patients with severe impairment of internal and external anal sphincter function and increased sensory threshold, training in synchronising both sphincter responses may be necessary (Figure 5).

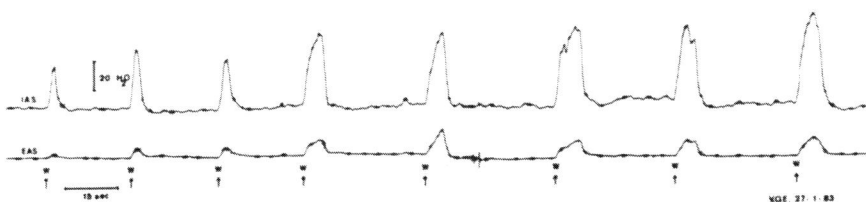

Figure 4. Manometric tracing from a patient with faecal incontinence. Repeated maximal voluntary contractions (w) of increasing strength during the first feedback session. Pressures are recorded by two balloons at the level of the internal (IAS) and external anal sphincter (EAS).

158

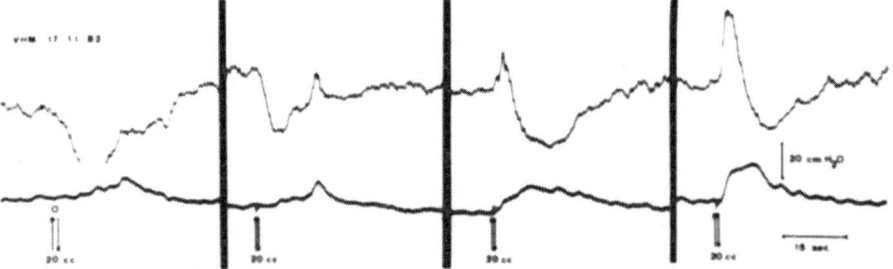

Figure 5. Progressive synchronisation of the external anal sphincter (EAS) contraction with the internal anal sphincter (IAS) relaxation to repeated distension of the rectum (20 cc) in a patient with a severe myogenic impaired anal sphincter during biofeedback training (F). The rectosphincteric response showed at the left was produced without feedback (O). Pressures were recorded with two balloons at the level of the anal sphincter.

Possible explanation why biofeedback is effective

There is evidence that every striated muscle has latent motor units which can become activated with exercise to the point that the muscle again becomes useful [10, 11]. The observations of Whitehead et al. suggesting that the external sphincter contraction induced by rectal distension is not a reflex but an automatic voluntary response, help to explain why biofeedback is effective in the treatment of faecal incontinence [9]. According to these investigators patients can learn to make a striated voluntary muscle response via alternative neural pathways, following an injury which interrupts the pathways normally mediating the voluntary response. It is known that voluntary responses, in contrast to true reflex responses, are less dependent on specific neural pathways. Furthermore, it has been demonstrated that the external anal sphincter is innervated by different efferent pathways and that there are receptors in the rectum as well as in the levator ani muscles [12–15]. These data suggest that, in patients with incontinence due to peripheral nerve injury, biofeedback may enable them to learn an external sphincter contraction response to rectal distension by facilitation [9].

Component analysis

Component analysis of biofeedback in faecal incontinence indicates that the mechanism of action of the three components of biofeedback training is complex and that not all subjects require all the components of the training for a successful outcome [16]. Manometric studies before and after feedback training demonstrated that this procedure decreases the threshold for rectal sensation and increases the amplitude of the external sphincter contraction. The morphology of the recto-sphincteric responses to rectal distension however, remain unaltered despite successful treatment [9, 16]. Conventional sphincter exercises without feedback do not improve the clinical condition of the patients [7, 10, 16]. An occasional patient improves without treatment indicating that biofeedback training is like all other treatment susceptible to expectancy effects [16]. Most patients respond to exercise training or sensory discrimination training alone. A minority of the patients require the classically described complex biofeedback procedure, including synchronisation training together with other training. The analysis of Whitehead and collaborators suggests that in the future it will probably be possible to make patient-directed treatment decisions.

Organisation of classical biofeedback training

During the training sessions the technique of ano-rectal manometry is used. The patient is positioned in such a way that the manometric tracing is easily observed. The subject who learns goes through three phases [1] (Table 1). During phase one, the severity of impairment of the rectosphincteric reflex is determined and the nature of the normal reflexes is explained. A good procedure is to show the patient a normal manometric record and to explain how his configuration differs from the normal. During phase two the subject is first conditioned to appreciate graded amounts of rectal distension in order to affect sensory awareness of the stimulus. Consequently he is requested to squeeze the external sphincter whenever he feels the distension or when he observes the associated relaxation of the internal anal sphincter. The pressure recordings are observed by the patient to help increase the amplitude of the voluntary sphincter contraction and to help synchronise external sphincter contraction with internal sphincter relaxation. Correct responses are rewarded with encouragement. Most patients who will have successfull training already produce a synchronous external sphincter contraction during weak rectal distension at the end of a single session. In phase three the subject is

Table 1. Phases of classical biofeedback training for faecal incontinence.

Phase I	– Diagnosis of sphincter impairment
	– The nature of the normal recto-sphincteric reflex is explained in detail
Phase II	– Actual training
Phase III	– Increasing amplitude and synchronisation of the sphincteric response
	– Generalisation training

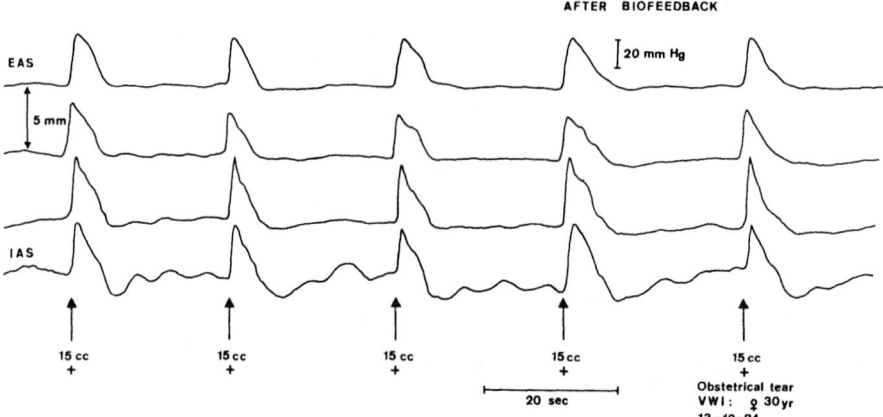

Figure 6. Manometric tracing of patient (V.W.I.) after biofeedback training. Normal internal anal sphincter (IAS) relaxation occurs with each rectal distension. The conscious sensitivity threshold is normal (15 cc). Voluntary external anal sphincter (EAS) contractions accompanying the relaxations can be clearly recognised. They are of sufficient strength to be detected by all the perfused catheters (distance between perfusion holes: 5 mm).

trained to approximate the amplitude of a normal sphincteric response (Figure 6). Furthermore, it is attempted to wean the patient from any dependency on the instrumentation. Therefore visual feedback is intermittently withheld by blocking the patient's view of the tracing. After a series of trials the patient is again permitted to observe his performance. After completion of the session the patient is requested to employ the learned technique whenever he feels the slightest sensation of rectal distension and to produce contractions four times a day for five minutes. One to five sessions of 45 to 60 minutes are usually required. During each session the subject is given between 50 and 100 trials with and without providing feedback.

Indications for feedback

Biofeedback training has been given for different medical and surgical conditions associated with incontinence (Table 2). It is also considered a modality in the management of children with faecal incontinence caused by imperforate anus surgery in infancy, longstanding functional megarectum and by spina bifida [17–19]. Patients with important loss of sensation for rectal distension are not likely to respond to biofeedback conditioning as they can not feel the urge that informs them when to produce the sphincter contraction [7, 17, 19, 20]. Elderly patients with dementia and very young children who are unable to remain attentive and to follow directions can not be trained with feedback [7, 17]. Depression in the elderly is not always a predictor of a poor outcome [7].

In general operant conditioning can not be applied in patients with painful active ano-rectal lesions, in patients with impaired intelligence who do not have the abilities to comprehend the procedure and in those lacking motivation.

Outcome

Biofeedback is a simple and effective treatment for different types of faecal incontinence even for those with slight to moderate impairment of the afferent nerve pathways. It has been applied with success to patients of all ages, including children and geriatric patients [1, 7, 17–19]. For evaluating the results of biofeedback training in patients with chronic faecal incontinence the rigid criteria for improvement, proposed by Cerulli et al. [20] were applied by most authors. A good response was defined as complete disappearance of inconti-

Table 2. Types of surgery and medical disorders associated with faecal incontinence successfully treated by biofeedback training.

Surgery
1. Haemorrhoidectomy
2. Fistulectomy
3. Fissurectomy
4. Perineal abscess drainage
5. Sphincter repair
6. Anal dilatation
7. Rectal prolapse repair
8. Benign anal tumour removal
9. Excision squamous carcinoma
10. Anal dilatation
11. Laminectomy
12. Meningomyelocele
13. Imperforate anus
14. Proctectomy for tumour

Medical disorders
1. Inactive
2. Irritable bowel syndrome
3. Radiation proctitis
4. Lumbar spondylitis with cord compression
5. Multiple sclerosis
6. Diabetic polyneuropathy
7. Cerebrovascular disease
8. Idiopathic faecal incontinence
9. Functional megacolon with soiling in children
10. Diarrhoea

nence or at least 90% decrease in the frequency of the incontinence. The overall reported success rate of biofeedback conditioning ranges from 50 to 95% [1, 7, 10, 16–20]. These differences may in part be due to different degrees of selection of the patients included in the reported series and to the different types of faecal incontinence treated. Data on concomitant aggravating factors in incontinence such as diarrhoea are lacking in most patient series. The results of comparable series including those of Cerulli et al. Goldenberg et al. and Coremans et al. are very similar. Cerulli et al. reported a large series of 50 patients of whom 72% showed significant improvement [20]. Goldenberg et al. obtained good results in ten of 12 (83%) selected patients. Satisfactory results were obtained in 13 of 17 (76%) of our patients (unpublished data). All these patients received conventional three stage biofeedback training as proposed by Engel and coworkers [1]. MacLeod reported a success rate of 72%, a percentage identical to that of Cerulli et al. [20]. The feedback training given to his 50 patients with faecal incontinence however, was limited to sphincter exercise training only, without additional sensory discrimination training. Biofeedback was provided by recording the electrical impulses produced by sphincter contractions which could be presented to the patient as an audible sound. The effectiveness of biofeedback training varies with the cause of the impaired anal sphincter function [20]. The best results are obtained in patients with myogenic lesions of the anal sphincters secondary to surgery. Less good results are reported in patients with faecal incontinence associated to medical diseases. In patients with gross loss of sensation for rectal distension due to spinal cord lesions the outcome is consistently poor. Of the patients in the poor response group trained by Cerulli et al. up to two thirds had severe organic lesions involving the afferent nerve pathway with loss of sensation as the results of meningomyelocele, diabetic neuropathy, multiple sclerosis and vertebral disc disease [20]. Follow up of the patients who had successful training shows that reccurence of faecal incontinence is rather exceptional [20, 21]. Cerulli et al. reported two of 36 patients who regressed within 22 months and required repeated conditioning which was successful. In geriatric patients progressive debilitating illnesses are most often responsible for a relapse [7].

Conclusion

Biofeedback conditioning in the treatment of faecal incontinence is a simple and cost-effective procedure. This technique proved to be effective for many types of faecal incontinence and provides hope for many patients with a socially and psychologically incapacitating disorder. Most of the responders improve after one training session. Up to now it is not possible to propose reliable criteria to predict with certainty a poor or a successful outcome.

Possible unexpected satisfying results, even in the apparently desperate cases, warrant a trial with biofeedback in all motivated patients able to follow the instructions.

References

1. Engel BT, Nikoomanesh P, Schuster MM. 1974. Operant conditioning of rectosphincteric responses in the treatment of faecal incontinence. N Engl J Med 290: 646–649.
2. Almy TP, Corson JA. 1979. Biofeedback – the light at the end of the tunnel? Gastroenterology 76: 874–876.
3. Miller NE. 1969. Learning of visceral and glandular responses. Science 163: 434–445.
4. Whitehead WE, Schuster MM. 1980. Therapeutic application of biofeedback in gastrointestinal disorders. In: Berk JE ed. Developments in Digestive Diseases. Vol. 3, Philadelphia, Lea and Febiger: 165–177.
5. Miller NE. 1974. Biofeedback: evaluation of a new technique. N Engl J Med 290: 684–685.
6. Colgan M. 1981. Medical uses of biofeedback: principles and case studies. N Z Med J 93: 49–51.
7. Whitehead WE, Burgio KL, Engel BT. 1985. Biofeedback treatment of faecal incontinence in geriatric patients. J Am Geriatr Soc 33: 320–324.
8. Whitehead WE, Schuster MM. 1981. Behavioral approaches to the treatment of gastrointestinal motility disorders. Med Clin N Am 65: 1397–1491.
9. Whitehead WE, Orr WC, Engel BT, Schuster MM. 1982. External anal sphincter response to rectal distension: Learned response or reflex. Psychophysiology 19: 57–62.
10. MacLeod JH. 1983. Biofeedback in the management of partial anal incontinence. Dis Colon Rectum 26: 244–246.
11. Bennett RC, Freedman MHW, Goligher JC. 1963. Late results of hemorrhoidectomy by ligature and excision. Br Med J 11: 216–219.
12. Bishop B, Gary RC, Roberts TDM, Todd JK. 1956. Control of the external sphincter of the anus in the cat. J Physiol (London) 134: 229–240.
13. Schuster MM, Hookman P, Hendrix TR, Mendeloff AI. 1965. Simultaneous manometric recording of internal and external anal sphincter reflexes. Bull Hopkins Hosp 116: 79–88.
14. Scharli AF, Kiesewetter WB. 1970. Defaecation and continence: some new concepts. Dis Colon Rectum 13: 81–107.
15. Parks AG, Porter NH, Melzak J. 1962. Experimental study of the reflex mechanism controlling the muscles of the pelvic floor. Dis Colon Rectum 5: 407–414.
16. Latimer PR, Campbell D, Kasperski J. 1984. A component analysis of biofeedback in the treatment of faecal incontinence. Biofeedback and Self-Regulation 9: 311–324.
17. Olness K, McParland FA, Piper J. 1980. Biofeedback a modality in the management of children with faecal soiling. J Pediatr 96: 505–509.
18. Shepherd K, Hickstein R, Shepherd R. 1983. Neurogenic faecal incontinence in children with spina bifida: rectosphincteric responses and evaluation of a physiological rationale for management, including biofeedback conditioning. Austr Paediatr J 19: 97–99.
19. Wald A. 1981. Use of biofeedback in treatment of incontinence in patients with meningomyelocele. Pediatrics 68: 45–49.
20. Cerulli MA, Nikoomanesh P, Schuster MM. 1979. Progress in biofeedback conditioning for faecal incontinence. Gastroenterology 76: 742–746.
21. Goldenberg DA, Hodges K, Hersh T. Jinich H. 1980. Biofeedback therapy for faecal incontinence. Am J Gastroenterol 74: 342–345.

3.7 Rectal prolapse

H.O. TEN CATE HOEDEMAKER & H.G. GOOSZEN

Rectal prolapse or procidentia is a protrusion of all layers of the rectum through the anus. The condition is found mainly in elderly women and it seems as if the incidence of rectal prolapse is increasing. This may be either a true increase in incidence or a reflection of a greater willingness of patients to consult with their symptoms. There is also an increase in incidence with age. The vast majority of patients are in their sixth, seventh and eighth decade of life. Rectal prolapse is rare in childhood and if presenting in children, it is usually associated with chronic straining or chronic respiratory disorders. If presenting in men, the condition is often accompanied with solitary rectal ulcer syndrome. In the Birmingham series five out of the total of nine men had a history of solitary rectal ulcer, and all patients were below the age of 50 years [1].

Aetiology

Children

Chronic constipation and respiratory tract disease are well recognised causes of rectal prolapse. In some youngsters chronic diarrhoea or rectal polyp may initiate rectal prolapse.

Adults

Causes of rectal prolapse in elderly women can be subdivided into four groups, pelvic floor weakness, rectal intussusception, psychological disturbances and anatomical abnormalities.

Pelvic floor weakness

Weakness of the pelvic floor is often found in patients with rectal prolapse.

Pelvic floor weakness may be the end result of severe straining during delivery leading to diastasis of the levator ani muscle or pelvic floor neuropathy [2]. This theory is supported by the finding that rectal prolapse is far more frequent in multiparous women. Rectal prolapse is however by no means confined to this group. The percentage of incontinence is about four times higher in multiparous women, suggesting the possible role of pelvic floor neuropathy as the cause of their disabling condition [1].

Rectal intussusception

Intussusception of the rectum is now considered an early stage of rectal prolapse. Although rectal intussusception, incomplete and complete rectal prolapse may represent different stages of the same disease process, there is no data from studies on the natural history of rectal intussusception to suggest that this develops into a complete rectal prolapse. These patients represent a different group than those, with pelvic floor weakness, since they usually have normal pelvic floor function and are not frankly incontinent [3].

Psychological abnormalities

Although some authors like Goligher [4] and Corman [5] have put emphasis on psychological aspects, stating that about 30% of their patients were 'rather odd' or even 'neurotic', there are no data on thorough psychological evaluation to support these impressions. Clinicians will query whether psychological abnormalities are the cause or a sequela of this embarrassing condition.

Anatomical abnormalities

A wide ano-rectal angle, a deep Douglas pouch and an elongated sigmoid colon have been proposed as causes of rectal prolapse. These features are more likely to be accompanying findings to a completely developed pathological condition.

Clinical presentation

Children

In children rectal prolapse is often incomplete and actually demonstrating a prolapse is not always easy. Differentiation from a mucosal prolapse, rectal intussusception, or a polypoid lesion may be quite difficult. The youngster is either severely constipated or chronically coughing and complaining of mucoid discharge.

Adults

The most prominent symptom is the feeling of 'something hanging out of the anus'. This embarrasing sensation is accompanied by bleeding, mucus discharge, incomplete evacuation or false urgency. Although Keighley [1] reports about 70% incontinence in patients with rectal prolapse, others have described constipation in 6–100% of their patients [6–17]. Sometimes there is also urinary incontinence. Pain is a rare symptom. On physical examination with the patient in left lateral position, perineal descent and a patulous anus are often seen, usually in patients with faecal incontinence. In these patients, during digital examination, the anal tone is lax. The prolapse can be demonstrated during straining and in longstanding prolapse, mucosal ulcerations can be seen either from repeated trauma or due to intermittent ischaemia at the tip of the prolapse. Sometimes, especially in patients with normal pelvic floor function, invagination of the rectal wall or intussusception can be palpated during digital examination.

Additional investigation

Clinical history and physical examination usually suffice to establish the diagnosis. Endoscopy and physiological studies can be considered in order to collect additional information.

Endoscopy

Sigmoidoscopy or colonoscopy are not particularly helpful in establishing the diagnosis but should be performed to exclude underlying pathology such as carcinoma or inflammatory bowel disease. It is important to realize that proctitis is quite common in patients with rectal prolapse and it disappears after successful surgical correction.

Physiological studies

Although patients with rectal prolapse and incontinence have lower maximum basal pressures and maximum squeeze pressures on anal manometry than those who are continent [3, 18, 19], no conclusions as regards the type of treatment nor its success, can be drawn from manometry data. There is considerable overlap between the two groups and the value for the individual patient is restricted [1].

Assessment of rectal proprioception or rectal compliance shows that threshold volumes are normal in patients with rectal prolapse. The maximum tolerated volume in patients with rectal prolapse alone falls into the normal range, whereas in patients with rectal prolapse and incontinence, the maximum tolerated volume is significantly lower than in normal controls.

Electromyography seems to be capable to demonstrate pelvic floor neuropathy [18]. We share the opinion of others that this type of investigation is technically demanding and not routinely useful. Defaecography is indicated in patients with clinical history suggesting incomplete rectal prolapse or rectal intussusception but has no place in patients with proven rectal prolapse.

Treatment

Conservative treatment only has something to offer in children. If they are constipated, behavioural treatment can be considered and in case of cystic fibrosis, medical treatment to alleviate severe coughing can avoid the need for surgical correction.

Surgical treatment

The only way to effectively treat rectal prolapse, if conservative treatment has failed, is by surgical correction of the anatomical abnormality that has developed. All patients should be offered surgical treatment since the disorder is embarrasing, especially if combined with frank faecal incontinence, and since there is a risk of bleeding. Several operations are available, all with low morbidity and mortality rates, if performed without partial colonic resection.

Rectopexy

Posterior rectopexy by the abdominal approach is the operation of choice nowadays. Although there are several important steps that need experience, the operation is well standardized and not a very difficult one. The pitfalls have been clearly described by Keighley et al. [19]. The documented mortality rates are low and rarely exceed 1% [4, 19, 20]. Fixation of the rectum to the promontory can be performed with Marlex mesh [4], ivalon sponge [21] or with non-resorbable stitches [4, 22]. The recurrence rates vary from 0%, to 3% and up to 12% respectively. From these data it is impossible to conclude which type of rectal fixation is superior, but probably fixation with Marlex mesh is most commonly practiced nowadays. Posterior rectopexy merely fixes the rectum and prevents further intussusception. Furthermore, the procedure has no influence on accompanying constipation, and its effect on faecal incontinence is unpredictable.

Resection

Partial colonic resection has been performed either as an isolated procedure to treat rectal prolapse or in combination with posterior rectopexy in patients with rectal prolapse and constipation. Recently Watts et al. [20] have advocated the combination of posterior rectopexy with sigmoid resection. Recurrence rates reported, ranging from 0–3.7%, are comparable to those of posterior rectopexy, but the series described are small. The addition of partial colectomy with end-to-end anastomosis to posterior rectopexy is however associated with a 4% complication rate, directly related to the anastomosis [20]. Of the patients developing these complications 50% needed further surgery. Although the results of posterior rectopexy with partial colectomy are encouraging, the approach to combine posterior rectopexy with high fibre diet and laxatives seems more rational, and maybe the patients that had undergone combined surgical treatment would have fared equally well with rectopexy only. This is also safer since resection and introduction of a foreign body behind the rectum considerably increases the risk of implant sepsis.

Rectal prolapse is associated with faecal incontinence in 11 to 81% of patients [20]. It has not been resolved whether the presence of the rectal prolapse can have caused faecal incontinence or whether this develops as a result of the underlying disease. In patients with the descending perineum syndrome having low anal resting and squeeze pressures, abnormal EMG recordings and abnormal pudendal nerve latency studies, rectal prolapse is found in only a few patients [23]. Both incontinence and prolapse of the rectum may be manifestations of the underlying neurological disease process. Neill et al. [18] supported the view of the rectal prolapse and faecal incontinence being secondary to denervation of the pelvic floor. It is striking that only a small proportion of patients with low spinal lesions develop rectal prolapse [24].

For some unknown reason about 50% of patients undergoing posterior rectopexy for rectal prolapse associated with faecal incontinence, are fully continent after operation [20]. If subsequent post-anal repair is performed in patients who are still incontinent after posterior rectopexy, 80% of these regain continence. So in the end in 90% of patients with the combination of rectal prolapse and faecal incontinence, the anatomical defect and continence can be restored. It is impossible to predict which patients will respond to posterior rectopexy only and who will need combined surgical treatment. It is therefore widely accepted in patients with rectal prolapse and faecal incontinence to perform posterior rectopexy first and to add post-anal repair at a later stage if faecal incontinence persists.

Post-anal repair

Post-anal repair of the pelvic floor muscles can be performed transabdominally or from below through the perineum. The results of the combination of posterior rectopexy with post-anal repair have been discussed above. There are also reports in the literature of the effect of post-anal repair only on rectal prolapse. The transabdominal approach is difficult as compared to the post-anal repair through the perineum. Pelvic floor repair for rectal prolapse is theoretically not an appealing operation for those patients with rectal prolapse and normal pelvic floor function. The approach seems to be insufficient in elderly women with documented pelvic floor weakness, as shown in reports in the literature describing recurrence percentages from 6 to 48% [1]. These reports, however, date back to the era when no manometry equipment was available and the patients studied could not be divided into those with and without normal pelvic floor function.

Peri-anal suture

The peri-anal suture for the treatment of rectal prolapse has been almost completely abandoned. In some patients it succeeds in preventing the rectum to prolapse, but it can aggravate symptoms like constipation, incomplete evacuation, and false urgency. Recurrence percentages are high (up to 67%) [1, 25] and there is a substantial risk of local infection. More recently described techniques suggesting the insertion of silicone rubber bands around the rectum above the levator ani and two around the anal canal may give better results in treating rectal prolapse [24] but theoretically there are serious disadvantages. The prosthesis can migrate into the rectum possibly leading to pelvic sepsis, particularly in case of recurrent rectal prolapse. Another complication is stenosis because the prosthesis is placed too tight, reoperation can be very difficult because of fibrosis forming around the silicone rubber rings. Similar experience has been collected in patients treated by the Angelchick prosthesis implanted for hiatal hernia or refluxoesophagitis.

Summary

Clinical history and physical examination usually suffice to diagnose rectal prolapse. Additional physiological studies are capable to separate patients into those in which pelvic floor weakness seems to be the primary disorder and those who have normal pelvic floor function with rectal intussusception. Both groups will undergo posterior rectopexy as the surgical treatment of choice. Patients who remain constipated will be subjected to medical treatment and patients who will still be incontinent can be adequately treated by post-anal repair through the perineum.

Literature

1. Keighley MRB. 1986. Rectal prolapse and its management. Progress in surgery: 114–151.
2. Snooks SJ, Swash M, Henry MM, Setchell M. 1985. Risk factors in childbirth causing damage to the pelvic floor innervation. Br J Surg 72 supp: S15–17.
3. Frenckner B, Ihre T. 1976. Function of the anal sphincters in patients with intussusception of the rectum. Gut 17: 147–151.
4. Goligher JC. 1984. Prolapse of the rectum. In: Goligher J (ed). Surgery of the Rectum and Anus. London: Balliere Tindall: 246–285.
5. Corman ML. 1984. Rectal prolapse. In: Corman ML (ed). Colon and Rectal Surgery. Philadelphia: JB Lippincott: 151–175.
6. Mann CV. 1981. Rectal prolapse. In: Thomson JPS, Nichols RJ, Williams CB (eds). Colorectal disease. London: William Heinemann Med. Books Ltd: 113–120.
7. White CM, Findlay JM, Price JJ. 1980. The occult rectal prolapse syndrome. Br J Surg 67: 528–530.
8. Hoitsma HFW, Meijer S, Klinkenberg-Knol EC, den Otter G. 1984. The treatment of complete rectal prolapse by transabdominal posterior rectopexy. Neth J Surg 36: 73–76.
9. Shafik A. 1981. A new concept of the anatomy of the anal sphincter mechanism and the physiology of defaecation. XIII; Rectal prolapse: a new concept of pathogenesis. Am J Proc Gastroenterol Colon Rect Surg 32: 6–14.
10. Ihre T, Seligson U. 1975. Intussusception of the rectum-internal procidentia: treatment and results in 90 patients. Dis Colon Rectum 18: 391–396.
11. Schoetz DJ, Veidenheimer MC. 1985. Rectal prolapse, pathogenesis and clinical features. In: Henry MM, Swash M (eds). Coloproctology and the Pelvic Floor. London: Butterworths: 302–308.
12. Biehl AG. 1978. Repair of rectal prolapse: experience with the Ripstein sling. South Med J 71: 923–925.
13. Berk G. 1979. Die Procidentia recti. Klinische Studien zum Rectumvorfall. Chirurg 50: 173–179.
14. Failes O. 1979. Rectal prolapse. Aust NZ J Surg 49: 72–75.
15. Veidenheimer MC. 1980. Rectal prolapse. Surg Clin North Am 60: 451–455.
16. Jurgeleit HC, Corman ML, Coller JA et al. 1975. Procidentia of the rectum: teflon sling repair of rectal prolapse, Lahey Clinic experience. Dis Colon Rectum 18: 464–467.
17. Nienhuis JE. 1983. De rectumprolaps. Thesis, Rotterdam.
18. Neill ME, Parks AG, Swash M. 1981. Physiological studies of the anal sphincter musculature in faecal incontinence and rectal prolapse. Br J Surg 68: 531–536.
19. Keighley MRB, Fielding JWL, Alexander-Williams J. 1983. Results of marlex mesh abdominal rectopexy for rectal prolapse in 100 consecutive patients. Br J Surg 70: 229–232.
20. Watts JD, Rothenberger DA, Goldberg SM. 1985. Rectal prolapse, treatment. In: Henry MM, Swash M (eds). Coloproctology and the Pelvic Floor. London: Butterworths: 308–339.
21. Boulos PB, Stryker SJ, Nicholls RJ. 1984. The long-term results of polyvinylalcohol (ivalon) sponge for rectal prolapse in young patients. Br J Surg 71: 213–214.

172

22. Carter AE. 1983. Recto-sacral suture fixation for complete rectal prolapse in the elderly, the frail and the demented. Br J Surg 70: 522–523.
23. Parks AG, Porter NH, Hardcastle J. 1966. The syndrome of the descending perineum. Proc Roy Soc Med 59: 477–482.
24. Todd IP. 1959. Aetiological factors in the production of complete rectal prolapse. Postgrad Med 35: 97–100.

3.8 Post-anal repair

N.S. WILLIAMS & N.R. WOMACK

Introduction

The post-anal operation was devised by Parks in 1975 [1] to treat patients with idiopathic faecal incontinence (IFI). The principles of the procedure are as follows. Under normal circumstances the angle formed by the junction of the anal canal with the rectum is maintained by the puborectalis muscular sling. The angulation allows the anterior rectal wall to act as a flap valve (Figure 1), and any rise in intra-abdominal pressure forces the mucosa against the upper anal canal and therefore effectively closes it. In idiopathic faecal incontinence the puborectalis is partially or completely denervated and this results in a widened ano-rectal angle and a shortening of the anal canal. As a consequence the flap valve mechanism fails to function satisfactorily and incontinence occurs.

Post-anal repair was devised to correct these abnormalities. By apposing the levator ani, the puborectalis and the external anal sphincter muscles behind the anal canal, the ano-rectal junction is moved upwards and forwards and consequently the anal canal is lengthened and the ano-rectal angle is made more acute. It should be realised that these aims are theoretical and there is some doubt, in fact, as to whether they are achieved in practice. Nevertheless, although there may be argument as to exactly how continence is achieved after the procedure, there is little doubt that post-anal repair can be very successful in many cases.

Indications

Patients with idiopathic faecal incontinence are best suited for the operation. The diagnosis will be made on clinical findings and should be supported by manometry and single fibre electromyography. A good clinical history and examination will ensure that the patient does not have another reason for

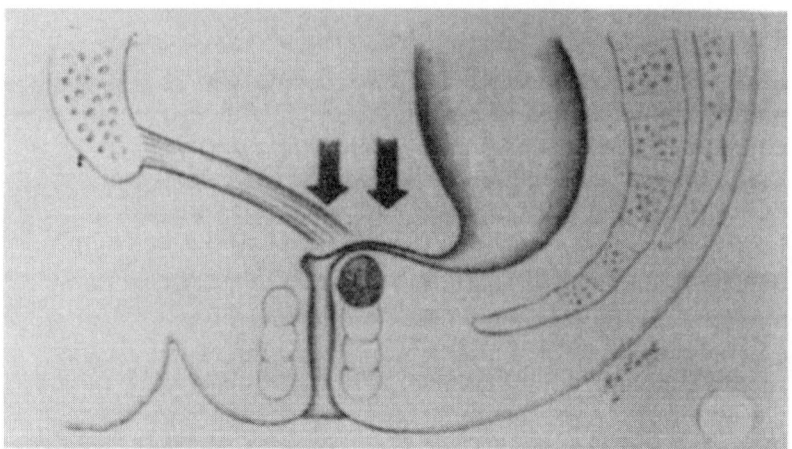

Figure 1. Flap valve theory of continence.

incontinence such as neurological disease, trauma to the sphincter or severe diarrhoea due to underlying bowel disease. Manometry will usually demonstrate a low resting anal tone (below 50 H_2O in our laboratory). Maximal voluntary contraction of the external anal sphincter will also be decreased. Measurement of fibre density using single fibre EMG should demonstrate a raised level (normal value in our laboratory is below 1.6), which indicates a pattern of denervation and re-innervation. Only those patients with severe incontinence who do not respond to conservative treatment should be considered for the operation. All patients should undergo a suppository regime prior to surgery. By ensuring that the rectum is empty of faeces at the beginning of the day, a substantial proportion of patients can be adequately controlled. Similarly, patients with IFI and concomitant rectal prolapse should have their rectal prolapse treated before post-anal repair is considered; in approximately 50% the incontinence will be cured by the repair. Although age is no barrier to the operation it is important that the patient is in full possession of his or her faculties, so that they will be able to co-operate with the postoperative instructions. There are some surgeons who will only operate on patients in whom the ano-rectal angle is wider than normal. As will be seen later, we do not subscribe to this belief, and, provided that the above criteria are met and the patient is fit for anaesthesia, either general or spinal, he or she should be offered the operation.

Pre-operative preparation

The patient should undergo a routine bowel preparation and we favour whole

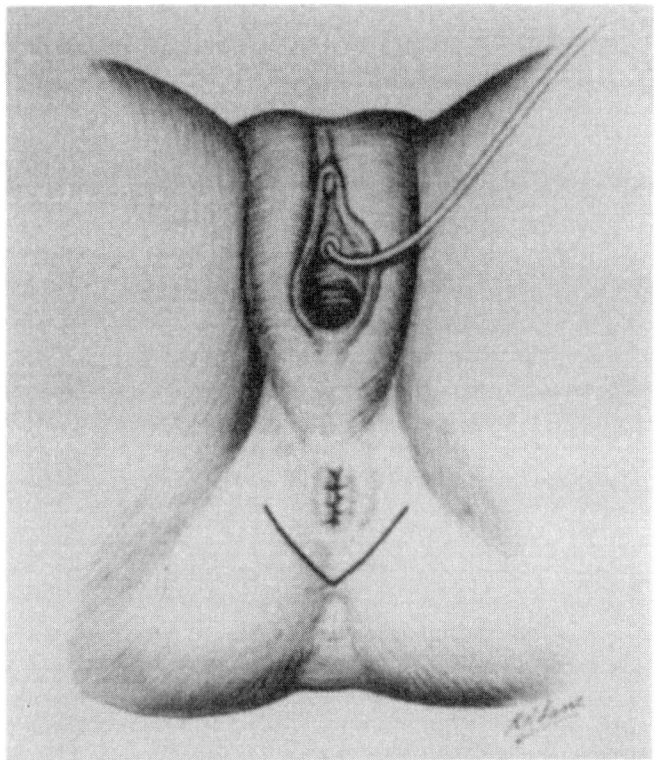

Figure 2. V-shaped skin incision for post-anal repair.

gut irrigation using oral Golytely. A three dose regime of prophylactic antibiotics should be administered. It is also wise to discuss the possibility of a temporary stoma with the patient, for although this is not a routine manoeuvre, occasionally it becomes necessary.

The technique

The operation is usually performed under general anaesthesia, but can equally, be undertaken with a spinal anaesthetic if necessary. The patient is positioned on the table in the lithotomy position and an indwelling urinary catheter is inserted. The subcutaneous tissue between the coccyx and anal verge is infiltrated with adrenalin saline solution (1 in 400,000) in the line of the proposed incision. Parks originally used a V-shaped incision with its apex based on coccyx (Figure 2). We, however, together with others [2] favour a more curved incision which is concave towards the coccyx. The skin anterior to

176

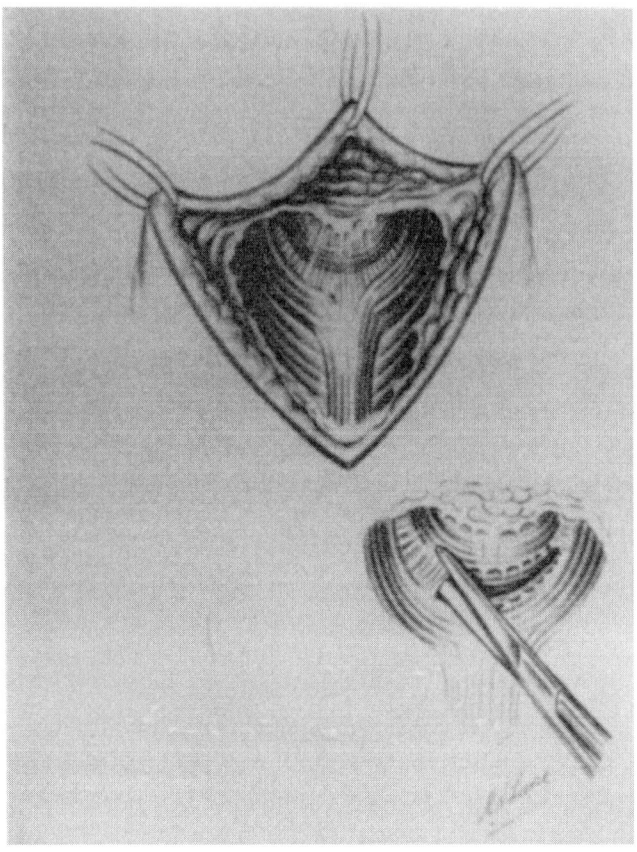

Figure 3. (a) The lower borders of the external and internal sphincters are displayed and (b) the plane between the sphincters is sought.

the incision is then raised with scissor dissection until the anal verge is reached. The lower borders of the internal and external anal sphincter are exposed (Figure 3a). The plane between these two is next sought (Figure 3b). This task is made easier by the fact that the external anal sphincter is identified by its red colour, whereas the internal sphincter is white. When, however, much of the external sphincter has degenerated, as is often the case in these patients, it is difficult to define the plane. Stimulation of the tissue with diathermy may help since this causes contraction of the external sphincter, but not the internal. It is best to start the dissection of the intersphincteric plane lateral to the midline. By gentle scissor dissection the internal sphincter is displaced from the lower part of the external sphincter through about half its circumference. The dissection continues upwards and is aided by displacing the rectum and internal sphincter upwards and the external sphincter downwards (Figure 4). Great

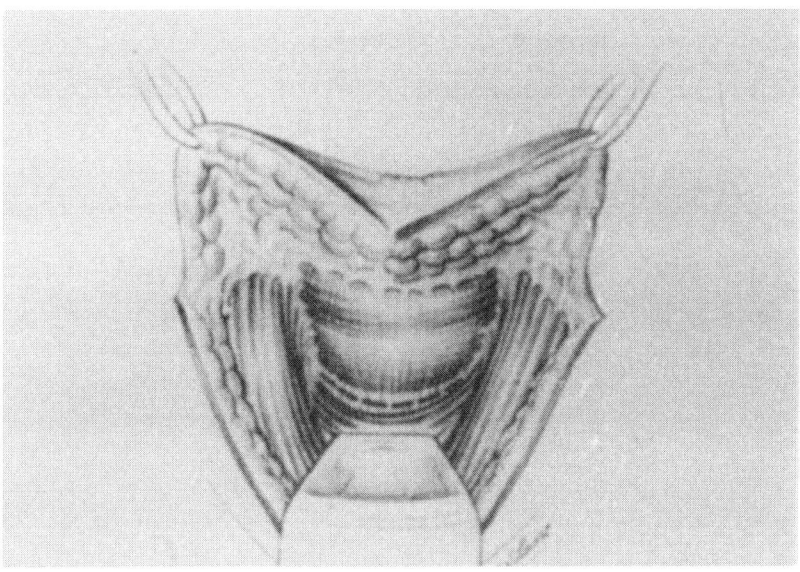

Figure 4. The fascia of Waldeyer is incised transversely, allowing access to the superior border of the pelvic floor muscles.

care must be exercised in keeping within the plane so that the rectum is not entered and the external anal sphincter is not damaged. It is important to continue the dissection as far forward from the anal canal as possible. The dissection continues upwards until the ano-rectal junction is reached. At this point Waldeyer's fascia is encountered where it is attached to the rectum and puborectalis sling. This fascia is incised close to the muscle (Figure 4) and this enables the rectum to be separated from it. This allows access to the superior border of the pelvic floor muscles. By suitable retraction the origin of the levator can be identified and the repair can commence. The highest and most lateral point of the levator group of muscles is identified with blunt dissection close to the ischial spine, and the first suture is placed taking a fairly large bite of muscle. The same is done on the other side. Three to four layers of sutures are inserted at this level, and they are not tied until all are in position. When tied, it is important that tissue is not dragged together under tension; it is therefore preferable to loosely tie these sutures so they form a lattice (Figure 5). The next layer of sutures is placed in the upper part of the pubococcygeus and again sutures are tied loosely to form a lattice (Figure 6). At a lower level, however, it is possible to bring both sides of the muscle together without tension. The third layer approximates the puborectalis and the fourth layer the external anal sphincter (Figures 7 and 8). A small gap is left inferiorly in both these layers to allow for any swelling in the tissues to occur post-operatively. A

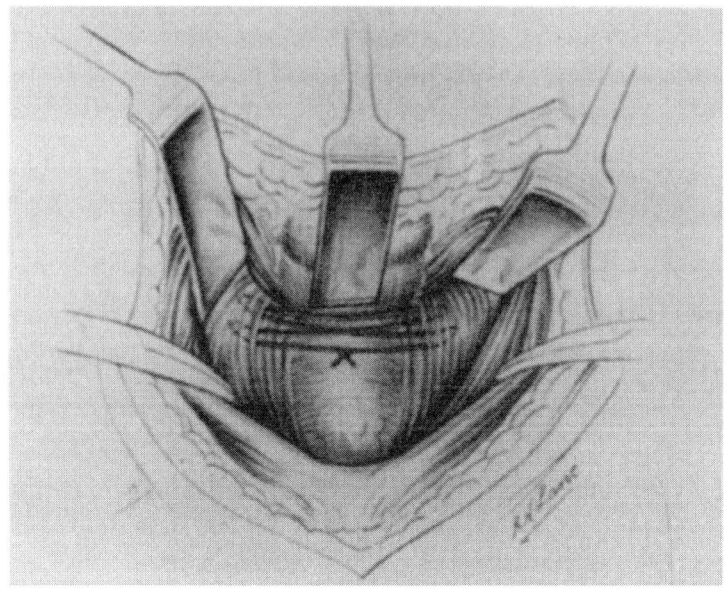

Figure 5. The levator ani muscles are approximated by a lattice of sutures.

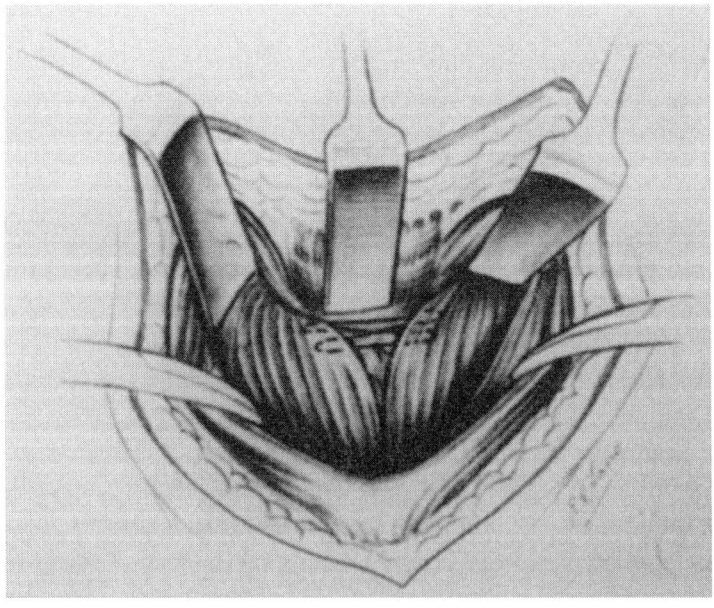

Figure 6. The pubococcygeus muscles are approximated.

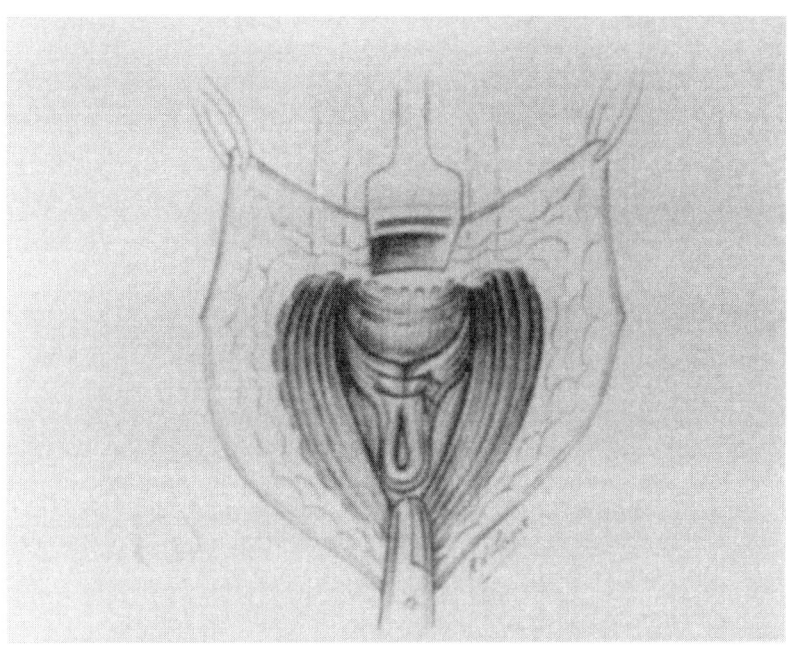

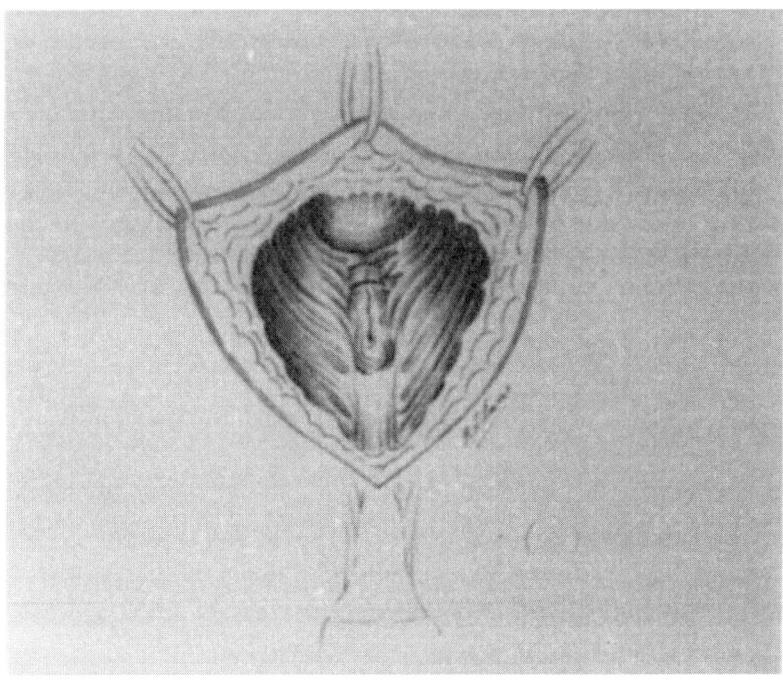

Figure 7 and 8. The puborectalis and external anal sphincter muscles are sutured together in the midline.

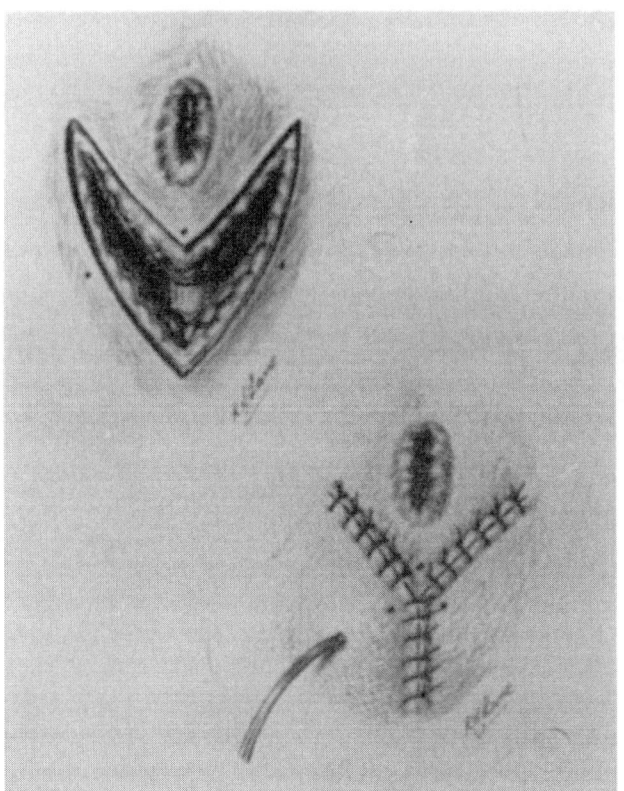

Figure 9. Skin closure is achieved by a V-Y plasty.

variety of suture material has been described for use in the operation; we prefer an O Vicryl suture on a small round bodied needle. This material is strong, yet is absorbable, and hence reduces the chance of wound sinus should infection supervene. The skin is closed over a small suction drain. A 'V-Y plasty' will be necessary for skin closure if an initial V incision has been used (Figure 9), but with the curved incision this is unnecessary. A covering stoma is not usually necessary, but if the rectum has been inadvertently entered during the procedure it is probably wise after repairing it to perform a defunctioning procedure.

Post-operative care

To prevent faecal contamination of the wound during the post-operative period we put the patient on an elemental diet for the first seven days.

Simultaneously, a stool softener, such as Isogel, is prescribed and also the patient is instructed to use glycerin suppositories each morning before rising. The aim of this regime is to ensure that the patient does not strain excessively on defaecation. This principle must also be carefully explained to the patient so that she understands that straining may lead to recurrence of symptoms.

Morbidity

It is not unusual for the perineal wound to become infected and for there to be some disruption of the skin. If, however, the patient has a good pre-operative bowel preparation, receives prophylactic antibiotics and is maintained initially on an elemental diet post-operatively, this complication tends to be of little consequence and usually heals quickly on a regime of salt baths. In the rare event of a major disruption of the wound a defunctioning stoma will be required.

Results

Of the 42 patients with IFI operated on by Browning and Parks [3], 32 (81%) were deemed to have had a successful result from the operation and 8 (19%) were classified as failures. Success meant that patients belonged either to Category A (continent of solid and liquid stools and flatus) or Category B (those continent for solid and usually liquid stools but not flatus). Keighley and Fielding [2] have reported on 40 patients who underwent the operation. Fifteen of these patients suffered from idiopathic incontinence and a further 10 had previously had a rectopexy. The remainder had the operation for a variety of miscellaneous conditions. These varied indications make interpretation of the results a little difficult. Nevertheless 27 patients (67%) were completely continent, 6 (15%) were improved and 6 (10%) were classified as failures.

Our own results (Williams and Womack, unpublished observation) – in 17 patients who each had IFI and were followed for a mean of 17 months are similar. Fourteen patients (82%) were improved at 12 months and can be categorised as A or B cases, whereas three (18%) patients were failures. It is important when assessing the results of this operation to take into account the length of follow-up. One of our patients for instance was continent at 12 months, but became incontinent at 18 months.

182

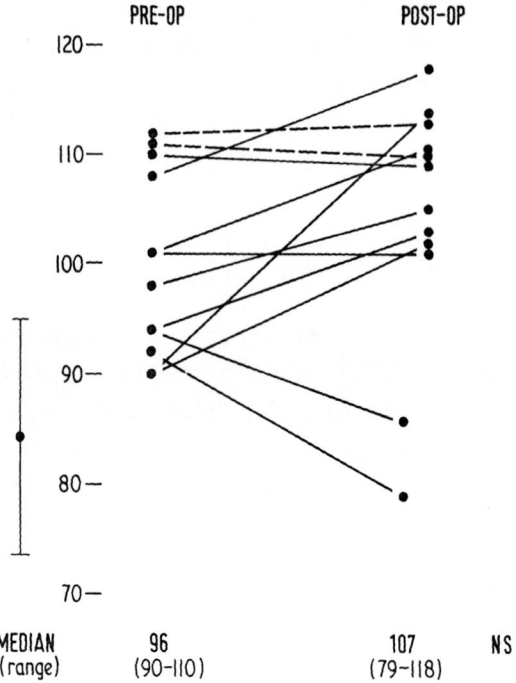

Figure 10. Pre- and post-operative ano-rectal angles – no significant difference.

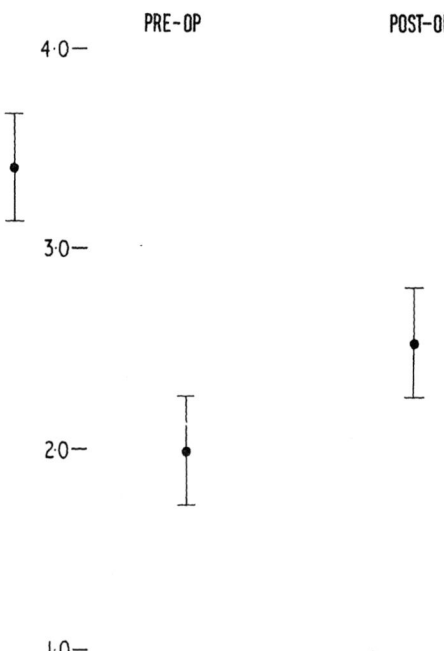

Figure 11. The 'anal sphincter' length was significantly increased after operation.

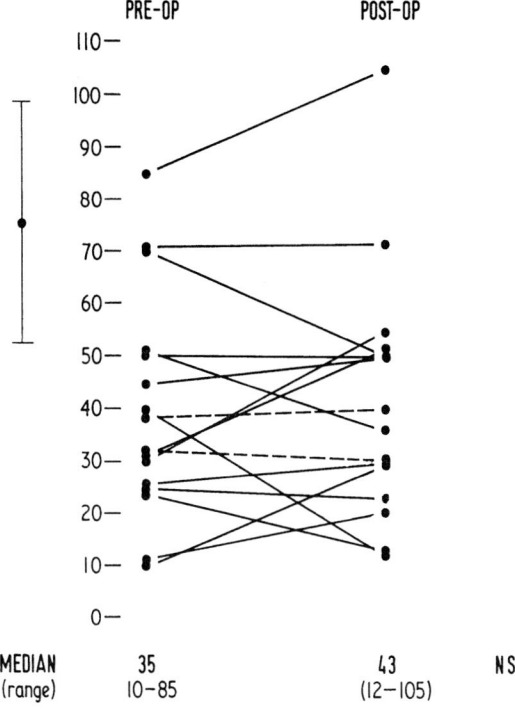

Figure 12. Pre- and post-operative basal anal canal pressures – no significant difference.

Physiological measurements

As discussed at the beginning of this chapter the operation is devised to decrease the ano-rectal angle and lengthen the anal canal. It is not clear, however, if these two objectives are achieved in practice. Our own study in the 14 patients who had a successful outcome following the operation (un-published observation) showed that the ano-rectal angle was not significantly changed (Figure 10). Indeed, many of the patients showed an increase in the size of the angle. Studies of the reproducibility of the method used to measure the angle showed that the error was too small to affect the validity of the results. Another important finding to emerge from this study was that five of our patients when observed pre-operatively had an ano-rectal angle which fell within the normal range and each of them had a good result following the operation. This therefore means that the size of the ano-rectal angle should not influence the decision to operate. We did find in common with other authors [3] that anal length was increased following the procedure (Figure 11). This measurement was performed using a station pull-through technique and,

184

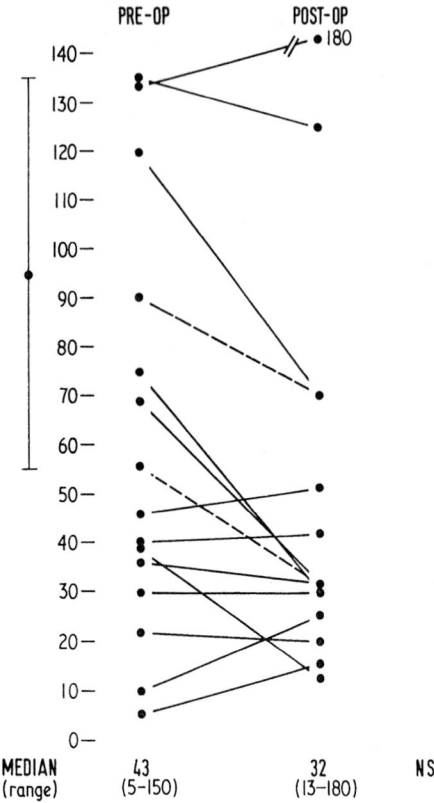

Figure 13. Pre- and post-operative maximum squeeze pressures – no significant difference.

although this change may be due to an increase in external anal sphincter length, it is not possible to be certain that this was the case. The change may be merely due to fibrosis which contributes to a high pressure zone. No matter what the explanation is for the increase in length of the 'anal canal', it appears that this is why the operation is successful, i.e. it increases the resistance to the egress of rectal contents.

Unlike other groups, we have been unable to demonstrate changes in basal anal canal pressures or voluntary squeeze pressure (Figures 12 and 13), findings which are perhaps not surprising. Basal anal canal pressure is generally believed to measure function of the internal anal sphincter, and the operation is not designed to affect this structure. Squeeze pressure is a measure of function of the external anal sphincter, and it would be optimistic, indeed, to believe that the operation would improve the efficiency of its contraction.

Acknowledgements

We are grateful to Miss J. Mutch who typed the manuscript and the Department of Medical Illustration and Photography, Leeds University and The London Hospital, who provided the figures.

References

1. Parks AG. 1975. Ano-rectal incontinence. Proc R Soc Med 68: 681–690.
2. Keighley MRB, Fielding JWL. 1983. Management of faecal incontinence and results of surgical treatment. Br J Surg 70: 463–468.
3. Browning GGP, Parks AG. 1983. Post-anal repair for neurogenic faecal incontinence: correlation of clinical results and anal canal pressures. Br J Surg 70: 101–104.

3.9 Sphincter reconstruction

M.R.B. KEIGHLEY

Introduction

We have used five principal modalities for the treatment of faecal incontinence. These have included control of bowel habit by anti-diarrhoeal agents as
a preliminary measure for patients with altered bowel habit [1]. The second
line of treatment has been to employ physiotherapy after a course of pelvic
floor exercises, faradism and a continence aid placed in the anal canal as well
as biofeedback [2]. Surgical treatment is confined to patients where there has
been no improvement in these two forms of conservative management. The
three principal methods of surgical treatment have included post-anal repair
[3], sphincter reconstruction [4] and a gracilis sling procedure [5].

Post-anal repair has now been performed on 118 patients by the author
between 1975 and 1985. Eighty-four, when reviewed at least one year after
operation reported that they were completely continent of solids and liquids,
twenty-one reported that they were continent with solids but not with liquids
and only 13 stated that they had been only partially improved. However, the
author would wish to point out that these patients were very carefully selected.
Post-anal repair was never performed early after an obstetric injury, was not
performed on patients with a complete neuropathy of the pelvic floor when
there was no recruitment on attempted contraction and the operation has not
been widely performed in the elderly patient.

Gracilis sling transplant has only been used on five patients and has been
confined to patients who have not been improved by other more conventional
forms of surgical therapy.

Sphincter reconstruction

Sphincter reconstruction has now been performed in 37 patients by the author
between 1975 and 1985. The results are shown in Table 1. We have reserved

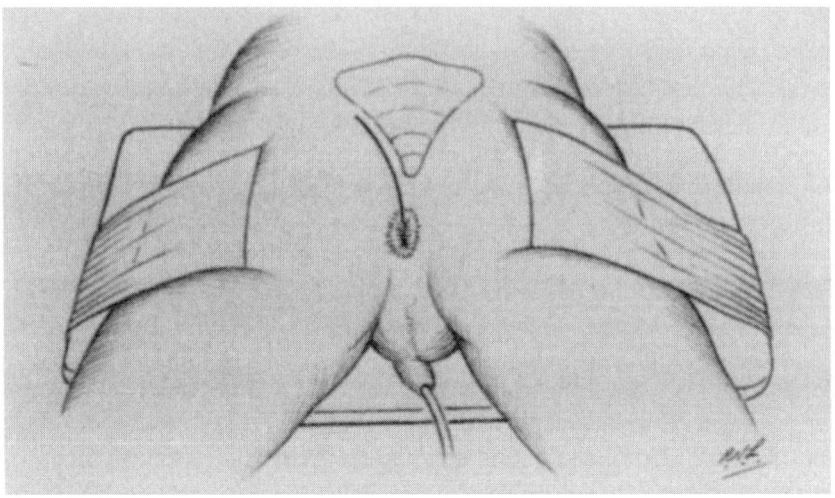

Figure 1. Jack-knife position in patients with a posterior sphincter defect.

sphincter reconstruction for patients in whom there is an identifiable deficiency in the external sphincter and where the remainder of the sphincter is
electromyographically normal. We prefer to avoid sphincter reconstruction
when there is any evidence of pelvic floor neuropathy and therefore exclude
patients for this operation if electromyography of the puborectalis is abnormal
or where the ano-rectal angle seems deficient on proctography.

We also believe that it is very important to insist upon a proximal stoma to
protect the sphincter reconstruction. For this reason patients must be prepared
to accept a temporary stoma if a sphincter reconstruction is to be considered.
In the past some of the sphincter reconstructions in our institution have been
performed without a proximal stoma and although many of the repairs have
been successful, if infection develops early in the post-operative period the
functional results are greatly impaired [6].

Table 1. Results of sphincter reconstruction (*n* = 37)

Continence	*n*
Continent of solids and liquids	29
Continent of solids only	7
Only partially continent	1

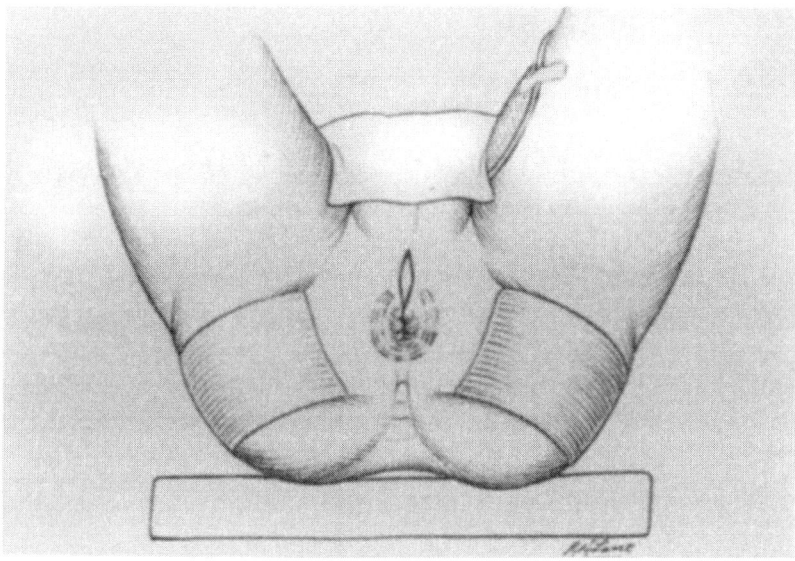

Figure 2. Lithotomy position in patients with an anterior sphincter defect.

Pre-operative preparation

All patients have a full mechanical bowel preparation. A stoma site is marked by a fully trained stomatherapist to ensure that the proposed site lies over the rectus muscle and that the siting of the bag is appropriate for the patient's normal clothing. We use peri-operative antibiotic cover in all patients, usually with a single dose of a long acting cephalosporin and high dose metronidazole. Patients are given a general anaesthetic and are intubated with full muscular relaxation. Anti-embolism prophylaxis is prevented with subcutaneous heparin or during operation by pneumatic leg bags. The operation is performed in the prone jack-knife position in patients with a posterior sphincter defect (the most common site if there has been previous fistula surgery) and in the lithotomy position for anterior defects (mainly in women with a previous parturition injury). The patient is catheterised and the buttocks strapped well apart in the prone jack-knife position with the table broken so that there is some hip flexion (Figure 1). If the lithotomy position is used the patient is placed on a sand bag so that the buttock lies well over the end of the table with a tray underneath the buttocks so that instruments can be placed in front of the surgeon whilst he is operating (Figure 2). The skin is prepared and the towels applied in the usual manner.

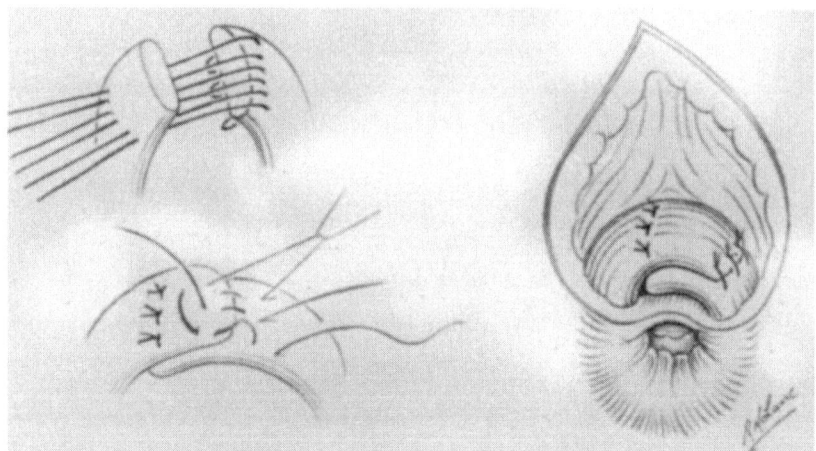

Figure 3. Deep layer repair in which each suture is placed and clipped before it is finally tied.

Operation

The mucosa of the anal canal adjacent to the scar tissue is carefully dissected from the scar and from the adjacent fibres of the internal sphincter. It is important to preserve as much anal mucosa as possible. Failure to do this will result in a fibrous stricture. The inter-sphincter plane is infiltrated with 1 in 300,000 adrenalin on either side of the scar tissue so that the external sphincter can be dissected free and a nylon tape is placed underneath the sphincter ring on either side once it is freed from the skin and from the internal sphincter. It is important to avoid excessive lateral dissection of the sphincter in order to prevent damage to the terminal fibres of the pudendal nerve. The fibrous scar at the site of the previous sphincter injury is divided in its centre. It is not resected since the scar is very useful in preventing sutures from cutting through the tissue in performing a repair. The mucosa is pulled caudally as the sphincter ring is flapped over itself prior to placement of the sutures. The deep aspect of the Mayo repair is performed first, each suture being placed and clipped before it is finally tied (Figure 3). Once the deep layer is completed the superficial layer is sutured to the underlying healthy sphincter as illustrated (Figure 4). The mobilised mucosa is then lightly sutured to the repaired sphincter but the skin defect is left open to drain. No drains are inserted and a small gauze pack is placed into the anal canal at the end of the operation and a dressing applied.

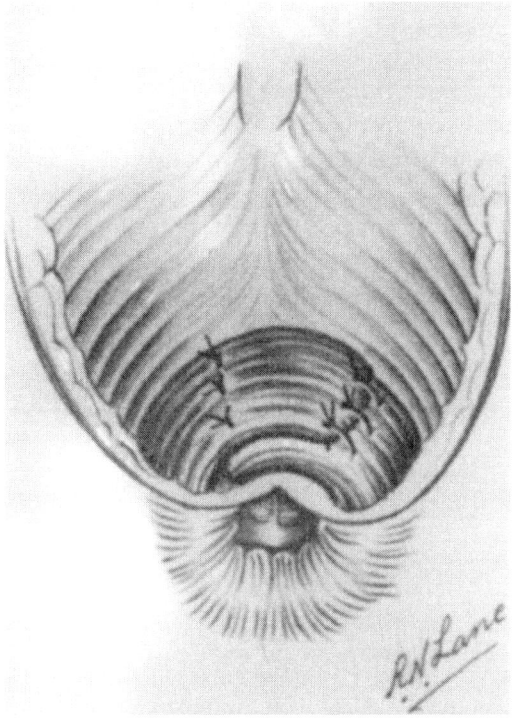

Figure 4. The superficial layer is sutured to the underlaying healthy sphincter.

Construction of proximal stoma

The towels are then removed from the operation of sphincter reconstruction. The patient is draped in the supine position and the abdomen is prepared and towelled in the usual manner. We do not perform a laparotomy for construction of a proximal stoma but merely excise a disc of skin and subcutaneous fascia over the marked site of the stoma. The rectus sheath is then opened by a cruciate incision and a cholecystectomy forceps is placed underneath the rectus muscle to facilitate diathermy of the rectus muscle overlying it, taking care not to damage the inferior epigastric artery and vein. The peritoneum is then opened by a further cruciate incision and the sigmoid colon is identified. The peritoneum on the lateral aspect of the sigmoid colon is divided to facilitate full mobilisation of the apex of the sigmoid loop. This is then raised to the surface, the colon is opened along one of the tenia and direct mucocutaneous suture performed without a rod. A stoma bag is immediately applied.

Post-operative management

The patient is maintained on an intravenous infusion for two to three days until the stoma is acting normally. The patient is then allowed small amounts of fluid and diet is slowly introduced after five to seven days. The patient is encouraged to mobilise as quickly as possible and if heparin is used for anti-embolism prophylaxis, this is discontinued once the patient is fully mobile. The patient is taught about the management of their own stoma and can usually be discharged from hospital on the 10th–12th post-operative day. We encourage regular baths to keep the perineal repair healthy and the open wound prevents any persistent collection of purulent material. Sphincter exercises are encouraged and the patient is seen by a physiotherapist prior to discharge for faradism and pelvic floor exercises. The catheter is usually removed on the third to fourth post-operative day.

Post-operative complications

The most important post-operative complication is sepsis. Fortunately this is extremely rare in patients who are given a proximal stoma unless of course the stoma does not adequately defunction the rectum.

Anal stenosis is another complication which may occur where there is loss of mucosa. If there is any risk that the patient may develop an anal stenosis it is a good idea for the hospital instrument maker to construct a small perspex dilator which the patient may use on regular occasions after their discharge from hospital.

If there is a deficiency above the sphincter there is of course a small risk of supra-sphincteric fistula. We have never encountered this complication but it may occur if excessive mobilisation of the sphincters is performed.

Results

The results of 6 independent series of sphincter repairs are shown on Table 2 [6–11]. Of the 195 cases reported in the literature, 137 (70%) achieved full continence of solids and liquids; 21% were continent of solids only, leaving only 9% who did not obtain clinical benefit from reconstruction. When we analysed our own figures we demonstrated that sphincter repair was followed by a very considerable improvement in anal squeeze pressures from 94 to 164 cm water but that there was only minimal improvement in basal pressures. We have no doubt that sphincter reconstruction is an important mode of treatment provided it is confined to those with an isolated sphincter injury and

Table 2. Results of sphincter repair (n = 195)*

Continence	Keighley and Fielding 1983	Browning and Motson 1983	Rudd 1982	Castro and Pitman 1978	Slade et al. 1977	Hagihara and Griffen 1976	Total
Continent of solids and liquids	24	65	18	8	16	6	137 (70%)
Continent of solids only	6	11	3	9	13	0	42 (21%)
No better	4	7	0	3	1	1	16 (9%)

* Reference 6–11

a normal pelvic floor. Failure to identify this group will lead to poor results. There is increasing evidence that many patients with a sphincter injury also have a neuropathy of the pelvic floor and under these circumstances we would prefer to use a post-anal repair as a primary procedure rather than a sphincter reconstruction.

References

1. Read MG, Read MW, Duthie HL. 1979. Effect of loperamide on anal sphincter function in patients with diarrhoea. Gut 20: A942.
2. Schuster MM. 1977. Biofeedback for faecal incontinence. J Am Med Ass 238: 2595–2596.
3. Keighley MRB. 1984. Post-anal repair for faecal incontinence. J Roy Soc Med 77: 285–288.
4. Parks AG, McPartlin JF. 1971. Late repair of injuries of the anal sphincter. Proc Roy Soc Med 64: 1187–1189.
5. Corman ML. 1983. Management of anal incontinence. Surg Clin N Am 63: 177–192.
6. Keighley MRB, Fielding JWL. 1983. Management of faecal incontinence and results of surgical treatment. Br J Surg 70: 463–468.
7. Browning GGP, Motson RW. 1983. Results of Parks operation for faecal incontinence after anal sphincter injury. Br Med J 286: 1873–1875.
8. Rudd WWH. 1982. Anal incontinence. Dis Colon Rectum 25: 97–102.
9. Castro AF, Pitman RE. Repair of the incontinent sphincter. Dis Colon Rectum 22: 290–292.
10. Slade MS, Goldberg SM, Schottler JL, Balcos FG, Christensen CE. 1977. Sphincteroplasty for acquired anal incontinence. Dis Colon Rectum 20: 33–35.
11. Hagihara PF, Griffen WO. 1976. Delayed correction of ano-rectal incontinence due to anal sphincter injury. Arch Surg 17:645–651.

3.10 Functional results after sphincter-saving operations for low rectal tumours

S. FASTH & L. HULTÉN

Introduction

Carcinoma of the upper third of the rectum (12–15 cm from the anal verge) is almost invariably treated with resection and end-to-end anastomosis. The operation is followed by an excellent functional result; except for a slight increase of bowel movements and urgency during the first post-operative months in some patients there are no differences as compared with the situation before symptoms caused by the tumour blurred the picture. [1, 2]. For carcinoma of the lower third of the rectum (4≤7 cm from the anal verge) it was long agreed that a sphincter-preserving operation is generally incompatible with the requirements of radical excision and until some 10 years ago tumours in the middle third (8–11 cm from the anal verge) were also in most cases treated by abdomino-perineal excision and a permanent colostomy. There were several reasons for such a policy: firstly, it was generally accepted that there should be a free zone of 5 cm distal to the growth; secondly, there was a very high rate of anastomotic dehiscence with concomitant pelvic sepsis after low anterior resection or rectal excision with a pull-through technique, which was at that time often used at construction of very low anastomosis; thirdly, the functional results after very low anastomosis were considered unsatisfactory whether it was constructed with a handsewn anastomosis by the abdominal route or with the pull-through technique [1, 2].

However, during the last years there has been a striking change in the attitude to the surgical management of rectal cancer in favour of a greatly increased use of sphincter-saving operations. The reason for this altered approach is to some extent that a safety margin of 5 cm or more is no longer always considered necessary, at least not in patients with favourable tumours where a distal margin of about 2 cm has been claimed to afford as good results as 4 cm or more [3, 4]. However, the main reason for the new approach is technical advances facilitating the construction of a reliable anastomosis in the deep pelvis. Such an anastomosis can now be accomplished by a stapling

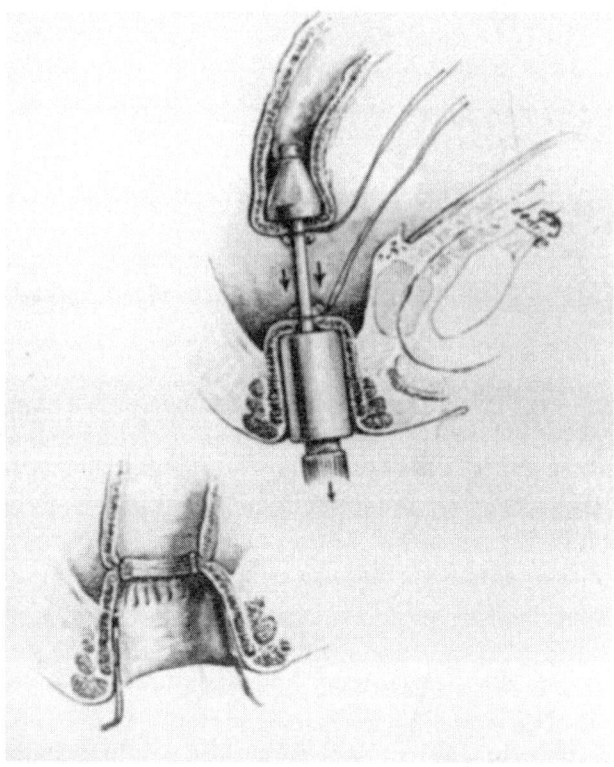

Figure 1. The end-to-end anastomosis (EEA) stapler permitting automatic suturing in the deep pelvis even after very low anterior resection which by definition involves full mobilisation of the rectum, partial or complete division of the lateral ligaments and division of the rectum at the extra-peritoneal part.

device, permitting automatic suturing at any level down to the anal canal (Figure 1).

Alternative techniques, either by an abdomino-sacral resection or an abdomino-transsphincteric resection, give good access to the deep pelvis, facilitating a handsewn anastomosis, but these methods are demanding procedures used mainly by a few experts [5, 6]. A further possibility is the abdomino-transanal resection with a hand-sutured colo-anal anastomosis, (Figure 2) a development of the pull-through technique [7]. The method has been recommended as an alternative to low anterior resection with stapled anastomosis and in cases where anterior resection is considered impracticable [8]. An important question is whether the change in policy might adversely affect the ultimate cure of the disease, a question that has still not got its definitive answer [9]. Another question is whether the functional results both as regards bowel habits and continence are acceptable after this type of surgery.

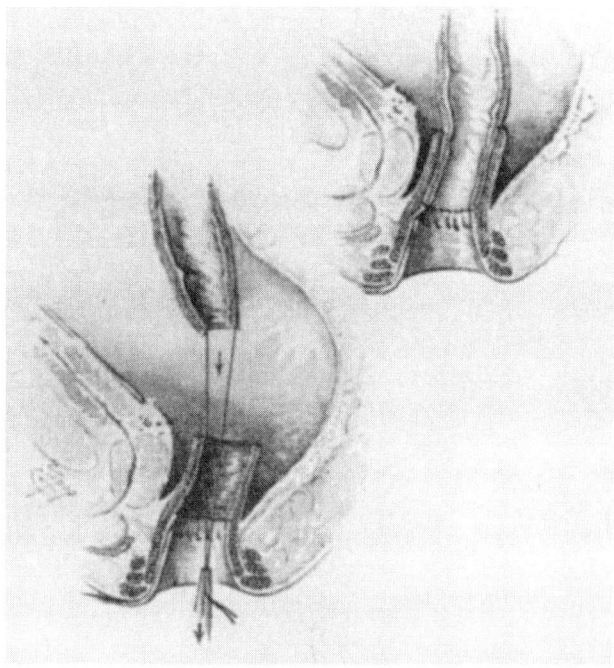

Figure 2. The colo-anal anastomosis is fashioned by joining the colon to the anal canal after removal of the mucosa down to the dentate line employing a peri-anal technique (7).

Subjective assessment

Colo-rectal anastomosis

In a detailed study on 32 patients subjected to a low anterior resection, which by definition involves full mobilisation of the rectum, partial or complete division of the lateral ligaments and division of the rectum at the extra-peritoneal part, Goligher et al. [2], reported that about 70% recovered full continence, but in those with a very short rectal stump (<7 cm) only about 25% could be regarded as having normal continence, corresponding to the bad results obtained in patients who had been operated by the pull-through technique. These ultimate results were preceded by a period of 6–9 months, characterised of considerably more pronounced disturbances with frequent bowel actions and severe urgency, coupled to more or less incontinence. By comparison the overall results reported in recent series with stapled ana-stomosis appear to be more favourable than those obtained by handsewn anastomosis in earlier series and several authors have claimed a fairly good function after a period of imperfect control [10, 11]. The reason why function would be better with the use of a stapling technique is obscure. However, in the early series the leakage rate with concomitant pelvic sepsis and anastomotic narrowing was often considerable, amounting to some 50% as compared to about 15% in collected series of later years [12] and it is probable that such complications might have influenced the results adversely.

The criteria of selection probably vary in different materials as indicated by a varying mean age of the patients which might affect the outcome as regards functional results. In our experience these are far from satisfactory when analysed in twenty unselected patients with a mean age of 69 years and with a stapled anastomosis between 5–10 cm from the anal verge [12]. During the first months the majority of the patients suffered from increased frequency, pronounced urgency and a good deal of incontinence for faeces and flatus. Although the function gradually improved during the course of 6 months, ultimately seven patients had still more than three motions a day and four patients suffered from severe urgency restricting their social activities. These disturbances contributed to the permanent disturbances of continence observed in about 50% of our patients. (Table 1).

The importance of the length of the recto-anal remnant has recently again been emphasized by McDonald and Heald [13], who showed that the function deteriorates as the anastomosis performed with circular stapling devices approaches the anal verge. For instance, the ability to discriminate wind from faeces and to defer defaecation was affected in about 50% of the patients with an anastomosis less than 5 cm from the anal verge as compared to 25% when situated between 5–10 cm.

Colo-anal anastomosis

The abdominal trans-anal resection removes the mucosal lining down to the dentate line and the muscle coat of the rectal wall to the level of the ano-rectal junction. From a functional point of view the collected experience after such an extensive resection and colo-anal anastomosis is still limited and the reported functional results vary considerably. Parks and Percy [8] claimed a normal continence in all except one out of 69 patients and similar results have also been reported by Rudd [14]. In other series the results have been less favourable. Enker et al. [15] found a disturbed ano-rectal function in about one third, necessitating enemas or laxatives to sustain bowel function and moreover many patients complained of urgency and of long delays in total emptying. Troublesome urgency, unpredictable bouts of frequent movements and a very precarious kind of continence whereby the anal control is apt to break down at a slight attack of diarrhoea have also been emphasized by several authors [6, 9]. It has to be stressed that these are the final results, not obtained until 1–2 years had elapsed. Due to local recurrence of carcinoma very poor results with deterioration of continence have been observed in patients with locally advanced carcinoma [16].

Colo-anal anastomosis with colic reservoir

The unsatisfactory functional results after very low colo-rectal and straight colo-anal anastomosis are an incentive to develop new techniques. Recently two French groups have presented encouraging results in patients operated with colo-anal anastomosis and 'J'-shaped colic reservoir [17, 18]. The frequency of defaecation was stated to be significantly lower in patients with a reservoir as compared with a straight colo-anal anastomosis and the continence was considered normal in all. These trials are in their initial stage, however, and it can be anticipated that a great deal of these patients will develop considerable emptying problems.

Objective assessment

Continence is dependent on a normal ano-rectal angle and a flutter valve mechanism at the ano-rectal junction. The effect of extensive rectal resection on the morphology is poorly known. According to Schweiger et al. [19], using radiological estimation, the recto-anal angle is unaffected by low anterior resection. A perfect continence is also dependent on a delicate nervous interplay between an intact sphincter musculature and a normal rectal reservoir, which are all affected by low anterior resection and trans-anal excision.

Loss of the rectal reservoir

Experimental studies with balloon distension have shown that the rectum is much more sensitive and discriminating than the colon. The quality of the sensation differs considerably causing a feeling of fullness in the perineum with a sensation of impending evacuation on rectal distension, contrasting to a purely abdominal sensation of colic referred to the suprapubic region at distension of the sigmoid colon [20]. These observations indicate that from a functionally point preservation of a rectal stump is of great importance. However, several studies have shown evidence that a colonic segment brought down in the pelvis to restore continuity after complete rectal excision acquires an imperfect sort of rectal sensation supposed to depend on receptors in the pelvic floor muscles [21, 22]. Pelvic sepsis and resulting fibrosis renders such an activation more difficult and may explain the unsatisfactory functional results after such a complication [16].

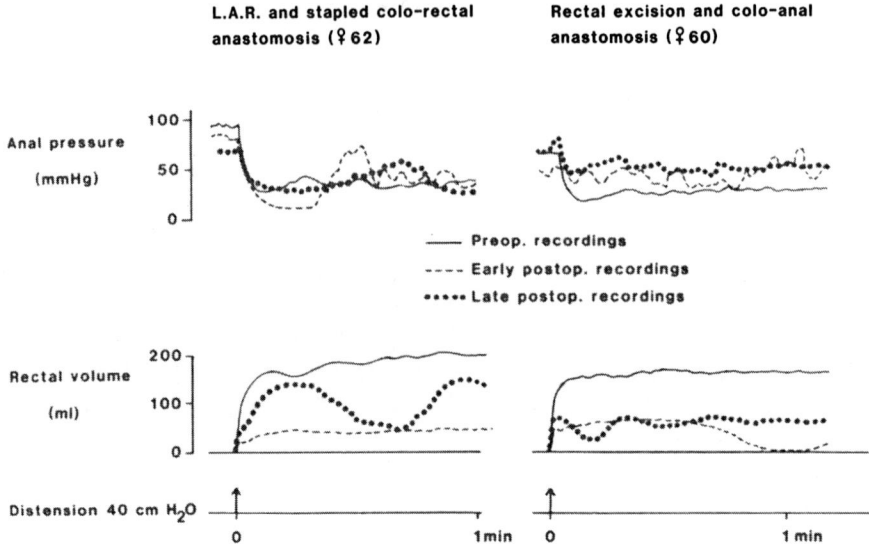

Figure 3. Dynamic responses to rectal or colonic (after colo-anal anastomosis) distension with 40 cm H$_2$O. Note the unchanged anal pressure response after low anterior resection and the reappearance of anal inhibition in the late post-operative recording after colo-anal anastomosis (dotted line, upper right panel). Note also the pronounced effect on rectal volume adaptation with a persistent low rectal capacity after colo-anal anastomosis and a restored but unstable volume in the late post-operative recording after low anterior resection.

Studies on the nervous control of large intestinal motility in animals have shown that there are specific fibre sets in the parasympathetic pelvic nerves which cause a profound relaxation of the rectum [23]. These fibres might explain for the ability of the rectum to accommodate to a sustained distension. This phenomenon is illustrated in Figure 3 showing the effect of continuous rectal distension on rectal volume and anal pressure before operation. After an initial shortlasting volume reduction (i.e. contraction) rectum slowly expands to accommodate the balloon used for distension and there are no further contractions. A corresponding distension of the descending colon after endoanal anastomosis shows a very marked reduction of the volume which does not noticeably increase with time (Figures 3 and 4). These experiments demonstrate the unique properties of the rectum subserving a reservoir function. As is shown in Figure 3, patients with low stapled anastomosis also show a diminution of the rectal capacity in the early post-operative phase. However, after 6–12 months there is a marked restoration of volume, but sometimes strong recurrent rectal contractions are observed. Such contractions that are experienced by the patients as a pronounced urge to defaecate are inhibited by atropine, and anticholinergic drugs have reduced the frequency and urgency in several patients, especially at night with concomitant improvement of con-

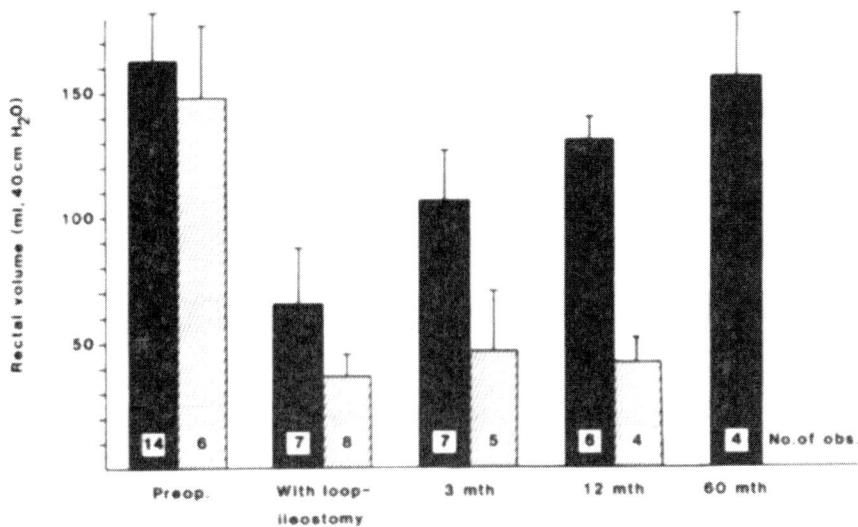

Figure 4. 'Rectal' volume (mean ± SEM) at intervals after:
low anterior resection ■
and colo-anal anastomosis ▨.
Note the restoration of the volume after low anterior resection contrasting to the persistent small
volume after complete substitution of the rectum with a colonic segment.

tinence. The persistent very low capacity of the neo-rectum after rectal excision and colo-anal anastomosis and the correlation between a clinical improvement and an increased rectal capacity with time after low anterior resection
have also been shown in other studies [16, 24].

Anal resting tone and squeezing capacity

The autonomous internal sphincter contributes about 85% of the pressure in
the anal canal at rest [25]. The reported effects of sphincter-saving operations
on the autonomous internal sphincter are somewhat contradictionary. Goligher et al. [2] showed a marked diminution of resting pressure in patients with
a short rectal stump (6 cm or less). The pressure in these patients was estimated to about 20 mm Hg corresponding with the pressure recorded in patients with idiopathic faecal incontinence [26] and incontinence in connection
with rectal prolapse [27, 28]. Williams et al. [22] also demonstrated a reduction
of anal pressure following anastomosis 3–7 cm from the anal verge, but the
levels exceeded those obtained in patients with idiopathic incontinence and
according to Keighley and Matheson [16] resting pressure is unaffected by low
anterior resection and colo-anal anastomosis. The external sphincter responsible for voluntary contraction appears to be unaffected after these procedures

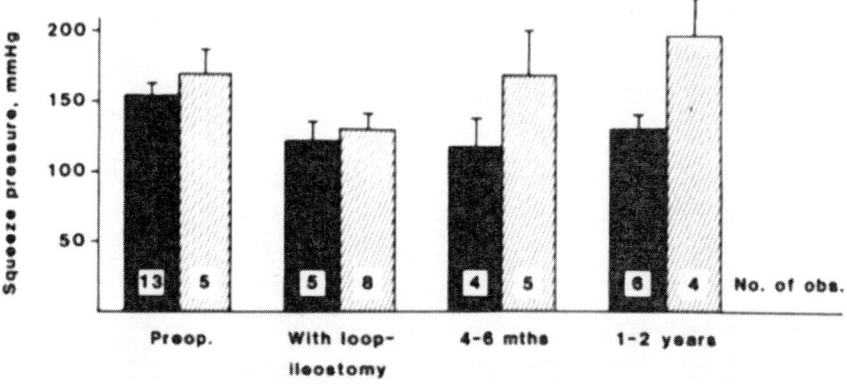

Figure 5. Squeezing pressure (mm Hg, mean ± SEM) at intervals after:
low anterior resection ◼
and colo-anal anastomosis ▨.
Note the increase of squeeze pressure with time in patients with colo-anal anastomosis.

[16, 19] and in our experience the ability to squeeze is even enhanced one year after colo-anal anastomosis (Figure 5).

Recto-anal reflexes

External sphincter contraction in response to rectal distension can be evoked in sleeping subjects, protecting against leakage of the rectal contents as the autonomous internal sphincter relaxes [29]. Prolonged distension is followed by inhibition. As judged by electromyographic recordings the reflex is intact both after low anterior resection and colo-anal anastomosis [21, 22].

Rectal distension inhibits resting anal sphincter tone [30, 31]. This decrease in tone allows the rectal contents to reach the sensitive anal mucosa allowing to distinguish between gas, fluid and faeces [32]. Goligher et al. [2] showed evidence that at least 6–8 cm of intact ano-rectum is necessary for maintenance of an intact recto-anal reflex. In our experience the reflex is intact after low anterior resection but disturbed after rectal excision (Figure 3). Lane and Parks [21] studying 12 patients who had undergone colo-anal anastomosis showed the characteristic response in 9, in some of them only after more than one year had elapsed, however. The observation that the recto-anal inhibition reflex may appear after a year or two has also been made in our own series of patients. This is exemplified in Figure 3, showing a profound relaxation before operation, absence of inhibition 1 month post-operatively and again a clear-cut relaxation 6 months later. The presence of the reflex is important to achieve continence after sphincter-saving operations [33]. The reappearance of the recto-anal inhibitory reflex with time might be part of the explanation for the subjective improvement sometimes occuring as late as one to two years after operation. It remains to be shown, however, if there is a correlation between the reappearance of recto-anal inhibition and specific function such as the ability to discriminate between gas and faeces.

Criteria for selection

The modern techniques with low stapled anastomosis or colo-anal anastomosis apparently give rise to a better functional result than the handsewn anastomosis or the pull-through operations used in the 1960s. Nevertheless, even in the hands of the experts in the superspecialized clinics there are still long term failures. Moreover, it has to be stressed that a function which is ultimately acceptable is in most cases preceded by severe disturbances during the course of the first post-operative year or even more after colo-anal anastomosis. Therefore the criteria for selection should be carefully assessed.

Tumour type

In view of the distressing disturbances during the first post-operative year a sphincter-saving operation involving a low anastomosis has very doubtful merits when life expectancy is short. Thus, in a patient with a low rectal carcinoma and distant metastasis for instance a Hartmann procedure with a well functioning abdominal colostomy probably offers a better quality of life. Moreover, although the curative value and the radicality of the operation is probably equivalent to that after abdomino-perineal excision the development of a local pelvic recurrence will give early and distressing symptoms that are difficult to manage and which requires abdomino-perineal excision within 8–12 months. Unfortunately, this operation, if possible to perform, will seldom be curative. Therefore a restorative operation for a low sited rectal cancer should be reserved for mainly limited growths with low grade malignancy and generous free distal margin below the tumour should be kept. Endo-anal anastomosis should only be considered for small tumours where adequate distal clearance can not be obtained even by stapled low anterior resection.

Intestinal function

Frequency and urge to defaecate, overwhelming a fairly normal sphincter musculature, appear to be the main cause of incontinence after sphincter-saving operation. Therefore the prospect of a good functional result is better in a patient with 2–3 bowel movements/week than in a patient with frequent movements. A history of irritable bowel syndrome, diverticular disease chronic diarrhoea (stool weight > 200 g) are other factors speaking against restorative surgery. If technical reasons or multiple tumours necessitates extensive colonic resection (line of resection above the left flexure) an ileal reservoir or a Kock pouch would be better option than low colo-rectal anastomosis, if the patient is young or refuses a conventional abdominal stoma.

Sphincter function

A patient with a history of anal incontinence, whether idiopathic or induced by previous anal diseases should not be offered a sphincter-saving operation. Elderly people have weaker anal sphincters than young people and therefore high age (>70) speaks against a sphincter-saving procedure. Disabling diseases like osteoarthritis, making it difficult to reach the toilet before the sphincter is overwhelmed, also have to be taken into account.

Whether objective assessment of bowel function and anal sphincter function with recto-anal manometry can be used to predict the outcome of a sphincter-saving operation as regards continence has not been settled. However, it appears reasonable to assume that a patient with a low anal pressure, although with a history of normal continence, carries a higher risk of developing incontinence than a patient with normal pressure and in our experience recto-anal manometry is a valuable tool to select patients most suitable for a restorative operation.

Conclusion

Despite all the enthusiastic reports as regards the functional results after the stapled anastomosis, the conclusion made by Goligher in 1951 [34] that to be absolutely sure of a normal continence an ano-rectal remnant of at least 7 cm has to be retained, is also valid when the EEA-instrument is used to facilitate the construction of a reliable anastomosis. When pre-operative evaluation indicates that a shorter remnant is necessary to ensure an adequate cancer operation (survival must never be jeopardized for functional benefits!) the patient is to be informed about the considerable risks for a disturbed function, even if a careful selection has been done before suggesting a sphincter-saving operation (favourable tumour, normal gastrointestinal function and normal anal continence). The functional results after colo-anal anastomosis indicate that if a patient with a favourable tumour, suitable for rectal excision and colo-anal anastomosis, is prepared to endure one or perhaps two years with severe disturbances the procedure is an attractive alternative to permanent colostomy in a physically and mentally fit patient. However, whenever a low anterior resection is considered practicable such a procedure is preferable to an endo-anal anastomosis.

References

1. Gaston EA. 1948. The physiology of faecal continence. Surg Gynecol Obstet 87: 280–289.
2. Goligher JC, Duthie HL, DeDombal FT, Watts JMck. 1965. Abdomino-anal pull-through excision for tumours of the mid-third of the rectum. Br J Surg 52: 323–335.
3. Pollett WG, Nicholls RJ. 1983. The relationship between the extent of distal clearance and survival and local recurrence rates after curative anterior resection for carcinoma of the rectum. Ann Surg 198: 159–163.
4. Williams NS. 1984. The rationale for preservation of the anal sphincter in patients with low rectal cancer. Br J Surg 71: 575–581.
5. Localio SA, Eng K, Coppa GF. 1983. Abdomino-sacral resection for midrectal cancer: a fifteen-year experience. Ann Surg 198: 320–324.
6. Mason AY. 1974. Trans-sphincteric surgery of the rectum. Prog Surg 13: 66–97.
7. Parks AG. 1972. Transanal technique in low rectal anastomosis. Proc R Soc Med 65: 475–479.
8. Parks AG, Percy JP. 1982. Resection and sutured colo-anal anastomosis for rectal carcinoma. Br J Surg: 301–304.
9. Goligher JC. 1984. Surgery of the Anus, Rectum and Colon. 5th Ed London: Ballière-Tindall.
10. Goligher JC, Lee PWR, MacFie J, Simpkens KC, Lintott DJ. 1979. Experience with the Russian model 249 suture gun in the construction of anastomosis in the rectum. Surg Gynec Obstet 148: 517–524.
11. Thiede A, Jostarndt L, Troidl H. 1981. Der Wert der cirkulären maschinellen Colon-und-Rektum-Anastomose (EEA: Eine prospektive Studie an 91 Patienten). Chirurg 52: 30–35.
12. Fasth S, Hedlund H, Svaninger G, Hultén L. 1982. Autosuture of low colo-rectal anastomosis. Acta Chir Scand 148: 535–539.
13. McDonald PJ, Heald RJ. 1983. A survey of post-operative function after rectal anastomosis with circular stapling devices. Br J Surg 70: 727–729.
14. Rudd WWH. 1979. The transanal anastomosis: a sphincter-saving operation with improved continence. Dis Colon Rectum 72: 102–105.
15. Enker WE, Stearns Jr MW, Janov AJ. 1985. Peri-anal colo-anal anastomosis follow low anterior resection for rectal carcinoma. Dis Colon Rectum 28: 576–581.
16. Keighley MRB, Matheson D. 1980. Functional results of rectal excision and endo-anal anastomosis. Br J Surg 67: 757–761.
17. Parc R, Tiret E, Frileux P, Moszkowski, Loygue J. 1986. Resection and colo-anal anastomosis with colic reservoir for rectal carcinoma. Br J Surg 73: 139–141.
18. Lazorthes F, Fages P, Chiotasso P, Lemozy J, Bloom E. 1986. Resection of the rectum with construction of a colonic reservoir and colo-anal anastomosis for carcinoma of the rectum. Br J Surg 73: 136–138.
19. Schweiger M, Schellerer W, Kuypers G. 1977. Kontinenz nach tiefer Rectumresektion. Langenbecks Arch Chir 343: 281–292.
20. Goligher JC, Hughes ESR. 1951. Sensibility of the rectum and colon, its role in the mechanism of anal incontinence. Lancet 1: 543–548.
21. Lane RHS, Parks AG. 1977. Function of the anal sphincters following colo-anal anastomosis. Br J Surg 64: 596–599.
22. Williams NS, Price R, Johnston D. 1980. The long term effect of sphincter preserving operations for rectal carcinoma on function of the anal sphincter in man. Br J Surg 67: 203–208.

206

23. Fasth S, Hultén L, Nordgren S. 1980. Evidence for a dual pelvic nerve influence on large bowel motility in the cat. J Physiol 298: 159–169.
24. Suzuki H, Matsumoto K, Amano S, Fujioka M, Honzumi M. 1980. Ano-rectal pressure and rectal compliance after low anterior resection. Br J Surg 67: 655–657.
25. Frenckner B, Euler Chr. 1975. Influence of pudendal block on the function of the anal sphincters. Gut 16: 482–489.
26. Read NW, Bartolo DCC, Read MG. 1984. Differences in anal function in patients with incontinence to solids and in patients with incontinence to liquids. Br J Surg 71: 39–42.
27. Frenckner B, Ihre T. 1976. Function of the anal sphincters in patients with intussusception of the rectum. Gut 17: 147–151.
28. Keighley MRB, Fielding JWL, Alexander-Williams J. 1983. Results of Marlex mesh abdominal rectopexy for rectal prolapse in 100 consecutive patients. Br J Surg 70: 229–232.
29. Scharli AF, Kieselwetter WB. 1970. Defaecation and continence: some new concepts. Dis colon rectum 13: 81–107.
30. Gowers WR. 1977. The automatic action at the sphincter ani. Proc R Soc Lond 26: 77–84.
31. Denny-Brown D, Robertson EG. 1935. An investigation of the nervous control of defaecation. Brain 58: 256–310.
32. Duthie HL, Bennett RC. 1963. The relation of sensation in the anal canal to the functional anal sphincter: A possible factor in anal continence. Gut 4: 179–182.
33. Iwai N, Hashimoto K, Yamane T, Kojima O, Nishioka B, Fujita Y, Majima S. 1982. Physiologic status of the ano-rectum follow sphincter-saving resection for carcinoma of the rectum. Dis Colon Rectum 25: 652–659.
34. Goligher JC. 1951. The functional results after sphincter-saving resections of the rectum. Ann Roy Coll Surg Eng 8: 421–439.

3.11 Surgery for incontinence and Crohn's disease

J.A. GRUWEZ & M.R. CHRISTIAENS

Introduction

Anal Crohn and incontinence are linked in different respects. Many gastroenterologists and internists advocate a very conservative treatment of granulomatous lesions of the anus, and many surgeons severely restrict the indications for surgical intervention or state otherwise that these lesions often end up with total excision of the rectum. Authors like Alexander-Williams and Buchmann [1, 2] state that 'often the only point in attempting to differentiate is that we should advocate a very much more conservative approach if Crohn's disease is suspected' while others recommend a conservative approach directed mainly at relieving the patient of his complaints [3–25].

There are some exceptions like Athanasiadis [26], Sohn [27], Lehur [28], Mareschal [29], Van Heuverzwijn [30] and the late Sir Alan Parks who performed some sphincter repairs in cases of peri-anal Crohn's disease. The major reason for this conservatism is fear for loss of continence. Unfortunately, such an attitude triggers a viscious circle permitting progression of the disease to a level where it can become destructive and definitively jeopardizes the continence mechanism. Another reason, or excuse for a conservative attitude, is the so called 'minor discomfort and indolent character' of these lesions. While most Crohn's disease patients do not spontaneously complain of excessive pain, they do find anal examination very painful. Moreover, nobody can be happy with a condition with continuous soiling, foul smelling discharge, irritation and burning of the eroded peri-anal skin.

We would be as enthusiastic as anyone in refraining from surgery in such patients if any medical alternative was available or if surgical treatment was ineffective. The message we would like to give is that anal Crohn's disease, even in its very severe form can be cured, and that sphincter repair can be performed in destructive types of the disease, avoiding any unnecessary delay in surgical treatment.

Present concept on peri-anal Crohn's disease

The experience we gathered during the last two decades in the treatment of Crohn's disease of the anus brought along a modification of our concept concerning this localisation of the disease.
1. Anal Crohn is a specific form of the disease and must not be regarded as a complication of intestinal Crohn.
2. The indications for surgical treatment of the intestinal form like abscess formation, fistula, stenosis, apply also to the anal form.
3. Previous surgical treatment of an intestinal localisation is not indispensable, nor will it induce cure of the anal lesions.
4. Surgical treatment of Crohn's disease of the anus is more difficult by the presence of the anal sphincter and the continence mechanism.

Patient material

The data of 121 patients with anal or stomal granulomatous disease, treated in our department between 1962 and 1986 have been studied. The male to female ratio was 69 to 52, with a mean age of 31.5 years. The total number of cases with Crohn's disease during the same period amounts to 152, which means that 79% of our patients suffered from anal lesions. In the literature the occurrence of anal manifestations varies considerably [31]. The very high incidence among our patients is due to their recruitment from a proctological clinic.

Clinical presentation

The clinical aspect of Crohn's disease of the anus can be trivial such as more or less complicated fistulas, fissures or oedematous skintags. Frequently however, a typical conspicuous polymorphous syndrome (Figure 1) with peri-anal dermatitis, intense oedema, longitudinal ulcers, abscesses and fistulous tracts, skin- or mucosal bridging, occasionally complicated by anal or supra-anal stenosis, is present. Carcinoma in anal Crohn's disease has been described [5, 7, 32, 33, 34].

Ano-rectal examination

The proctological examination of such patients should not be cursory. Spreading of the anus may convert a mildly abnormal appearance into a dramatic picture of florid Crohn's disease. Simple anal lesions were present in 49.5% of

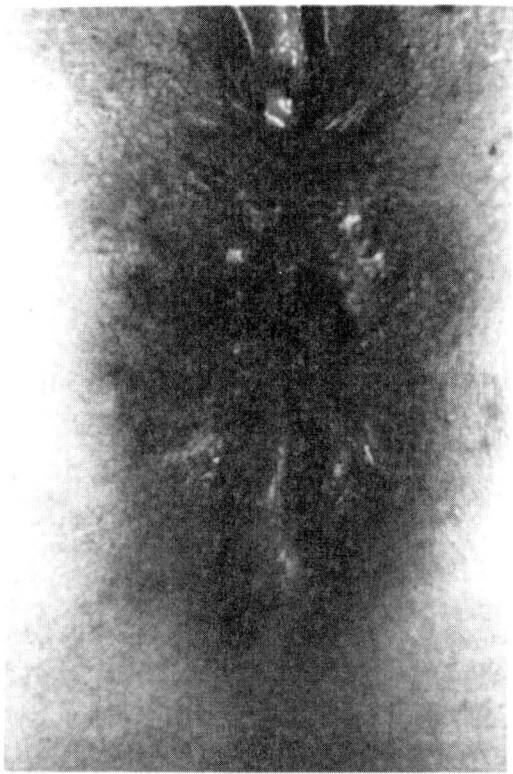

Figure 1. Crohn's disease of the anus: pathognomonic lesion.

our patients and pathognomonic manifestations in 50.4%. Thirteen patients presented with ano-vaginal fistulas and in 28 patients there was severe destruction.

Extra-intestinal manifestations

Concomitant conditions like erythema nodosum, arthritis and conjunctivitis or keratosis sometimes were present in our group. Evidently, clinical history, X-ray findings and biopsies are important in the diagnostic evaluation of such patients. The algorithm (Figure 2) illustrates how in the presence of an anal lesion Crohn's disease can be diagnosed:

1. A trivial lesion proves to be of granulomatous nature at histological examination.
2. A known intestinal involvement points evidently at the diagnosis.

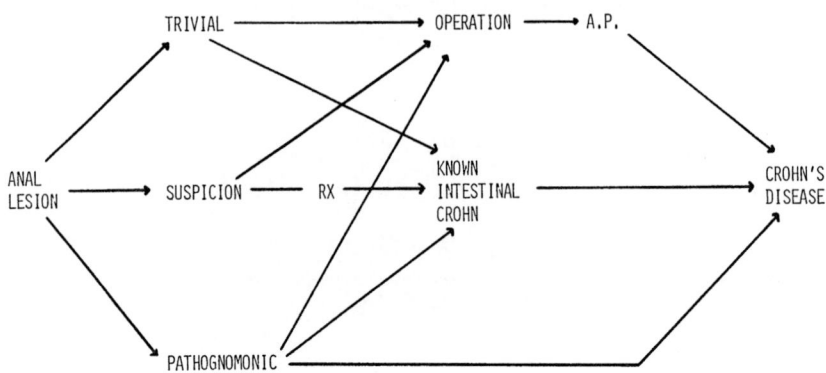

DIAGNOSIS OF CROHN'S DISEASE OF THE ANUS.

Figure 2.

3. The appearance of the anal lesion or the patient's history necessitates X-ray examination, subsequent endoscopy with biopsies and histopathological examination leading to the diagnosis.
4. Finally, the pathognomonic clinical picture permits immediate and unequivocal diagnosis.

The hallmark of the histological diagnosis is the 'sarcoid lesion', which consists of a Langhans giant-cell, surrounded by epitheloid cells without central caseation. As sarcoid granulomata are very scarse, histological diagnosis depends to some extent on the amount of tissue available. In 85 cases the histological examination was 'positive for or compatible with' Crohn's disease. In only 16 patients were aspecific inflammatory features found.

Although rarely, anal lesions can be the only manifestation of the disease (8 cases). 113 were combined with other localisations: 27 preceded, 41 were synchronous and 45 metachronous to the intestinal lesions which mostly involved the terminal ileum, coecum or ascending colon; 37 patients showed a diseased rectum.

Treatment

Our present therapeutical approach consists of:
1. Classical medical treatment course (diet, Salazosulfapyridine, Metronidazole [9, 35, 36], corticosteroids, eventually antibiotics, antidiarrhetic medications) and topical treatment (ointments – enemas – corticosteroids, 5-A.S.A.).
2. Surgical treatment:
– A simple proctological procedure: drainage of an abscess, syringotomy to take care of simple lesions.

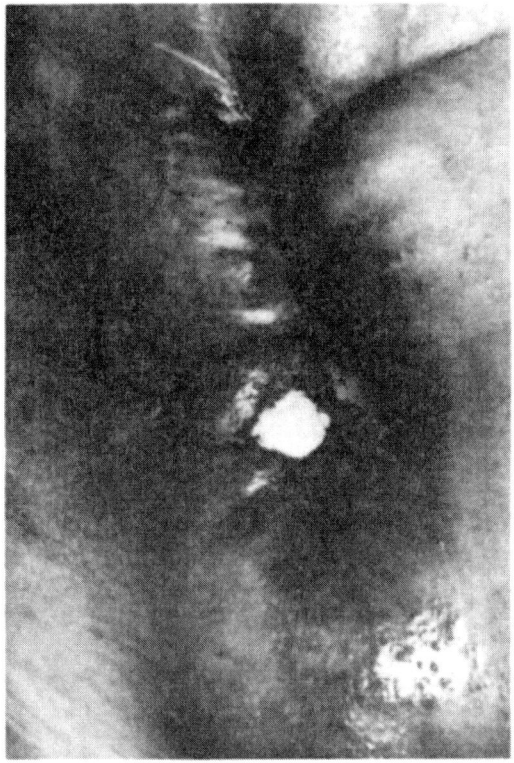

Figure 3. Peri-ileostomy Crohn's disease (a sponge indicates the location of the ileostomy).

- More complex destructive lesions, mostly the pathognomonic cases, need
  more elaborative, often multiple-stage surgical management: syringotomy
  combined with seton drainage, thorough debridement of skin tags, hyper-
  trophied papillae, mucosal bridges and fissures, curretages of granulomatous tissue, saucerisation and skin grafting if needed. A diverting
  colostomy or ileostomy can be necessary [14]. Meticulous post-operative
  care is mandatory for healing and prevention of stenosis (St. Marks dila-
  tors). Proctectomy has to be considered in rare instances.

In our series 63 simple and 56 complex procedures were performed. From our
results we are convinced that anal Crohn's disease should be treated at the
earliest possible stage and that an adequate surgical approach is in no way
more harmful than a conservative attitude. This policy results in improvement
or cure of the disease in 82.8% of our patients. In three of them a temporary
colostomy and in three others, a temporary ileostomy was necessary. Two
patients underwent coloproctectomy. Ileostomy and colostomy-fistulas were
treated successfully in two instances (Figure 3).

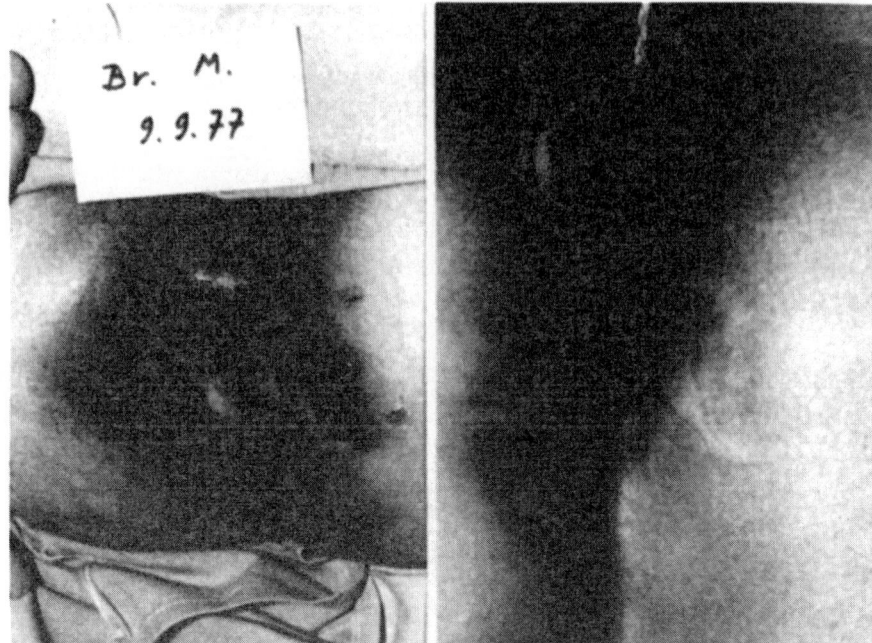

Figure 4. Destructive form of anal Crohn's disease and complete healing after thorough debridement and sphincteroplasty.

At the present time the treatment is still being performed in 17 patients. Four have a colostomy and two an ileostomy. One patient died after major intestinal resection subsequent to a peri-anal abscess drainage. These results can be compared with those of surgeons with a similar approach [28, 29]. They were never obtained by a more conservative approach nor by high doses of Metronidazole only [9, 35, 37].

Continence

85 of the 93 patients who are cured or improved are continent, five are incontinent for gas, three have faecal incontinence, mostly during episodes of diarrhoea. In Crohn's disease, as in many other conditions, anatomic disruption or destruction of the sphincter mechanism represents the most common cause of faecal incontinence.

Non-operative treatment or physical therapy have proven to be beneficial in alleviating symptoms of leakage and occasional loss of sphincter control, but fail when the sphincter mechanism has been destroyed.

Operative treatment aims at repair of the disrupted sphincter. Direct sphincter repair is the only technique performed. Sphincter replacement procedures (gluteus or gracilis muscle [38], prosthesis) or other operative techniques like anterior and posterior refing or post-anal repair can be applied but have not been used in our series. We performed 13 sphincteroplasties in 11 patients. Three patients are continent for faeces and gas (Figure 4). Four patients with temporary diversion, have developed a sufficient sphincter contractility at digital examination, manometry studies and retention tests. Three of them will have their colostomy closed at a later date. One has been admitted to a psychiatric hospital and will be lost to follow-up. In four additional patients sphincter repair has been performed too recently for adequate evaluation of sphincter function. In literature, data on sphincter repair in Crohn's disease are scarce, but the results decribed are comparable to those obtained in our series.

Summary

Anal granulomatous lesions should preferably be treated at an early stage. Even in destructive lesions surgical management can result in healing of damaged tissues, permitting sphincter repair in a number of selected cases. We therefore think that it is justified to be conservative for abdominal Crohn, but aggressive for the anal form of the disease.

Editorial comment

Clinical presentation of peri-anal Crohn's disease is usually not as dramatic as in the patients described by Gruwez and Christiaens. Quite often symptoms are mild and painful dermatitis only occurs during episodes of diarrhoea or reactivation of the disease. In quiescent Crohn's disease the proportion of patients having troublesome symptoms from visible peri-anal disease is less than 20%. [39]. Peri-anal fistula, fissure in ano and anal skin tags frequently disappear completely if left alone. Buchmann et al. [40] showed that 40% of patients with these lesions had a normal anal canal when examined 5 to 10 years after a diagnosis of Crohn's disease. Finally, anal dilatation for fissure and laying open of a fistula-in-ano was commonly complicated by persistent incontinence in the Birmingham series [39]. If surgical treatment is deemed necessary it should, if possible, be confined to drainage of pus under tension or occasional faecal diversion for severe cavitating ulcers or fistulas. The editors are rarely able to justify major surgery for fissure, fistula-in-ano or ano-rectal stricture. Crohn's fistulas do not respond well to routine procedures like laying open, curettage of granulomatous tissue or seton drainage. Such lesions tend to be much more indolent and do persist after surgical treatment. There is also a risk of rendering patients incontinent as a result of operation for fistula-in-ano. It is, however, acknowledged that some rectovaginal fistulas could with justification be treated along the lines presented by Gruwez and Christiaens. It is also agreed upon that some patients rendered incontinent can successfully undergo sphincter repair, provided that the disease is quiescent though a covering stoma is usually advised. This is, in our experience, only a minority of patients presenting with peri-anal Crohn's disease. It seems that Gruwez and Christiaens are confronted with patients at a late stage of their peri-anal disease.

H.G. Gooszen
M.R.B. Keighley

References

1. Alexander-Williams J, Buchmann P. 1980. Peri-anal Crohn's disease. World J Surg 4: 203–208.
2. Buchmann P, Alexander-Williams J. 1980. Classification of Peri-anal Crohn's Disease. Clin Gastroenterol 9(2): 323–330.
3. Buchmann P, Weterman IT. 1981. Peri-anal Crohn's Disease. Coloproctology. 3: 77–81.
4. Buchmann P, Weterman IT, Keighley MRB, Pena AS, Allan RN, Alexander-Williams J. 1981. The prognosis of ileo-rectal anastomosis in Crohn's disease. Br J Surg 68: 7–10.
5. Chaikhouni A, Regueyra FI, Stevens JR. 1981. Adenocarcinoma in perineal fistulas of Crohn's Disease. Dis Colon Rectum 24: 639–643.
6. Chapuis G. 1981. Progrès dans la chirurgie de la maladie de Crohn du colon et du rectum. Helv Chir Acta. 48: 805–812.
7. Daly JJ, Madrazo A. 1980. Anal Crohn's Disease with Carcinoma. Dig Dis Sci 25: 464–465.
8. Faulconer HT, Muldoon JP. 1975. Rectovaginal fistula in patients with colitis. Dis Colon Rectum 18: 413–415.
9. Frank MS, Brandt LJ, Bernstein LH. 1983. Pharmacotherapy of inflammatory bowel disease. Pharmacotherapy, part 2, 74: 155–172.
10. Gray BK, Lockhart-Mummery HE, Morson BC. 1965. Crohn's disease of the anal region. Gut 6: 515–524.
11. Greenstein AJ, Dicker A, Meyers S, Aufses AH Jr. 1983. Periileostomy fistulae in Crohn's Disease. Ann Surg 197: 179–182.
12. Greenstein AJ, Sachar DB, Kark AE. 1975. Stricture of the ano-rectum in Crohn's Disease involving the colon. Ann Surg 181: 207–212.
13. Gruwez JA, Christiaens MR, Lacquet A. 1983. La maladie de Crohn de l'anus. Acta Endosc 13(4): 285–292.
14. Harper PH, Kettlewell MGW, Lee ECG. 1982. The effect of split ileostomy on peri-anal Crohn's disease. Br J Surg 69: 608–610.
15. Hellers G, Bergstrand O, Ewerth S, Holström B. 1980. Occurrence and outcome after primary treatment of anal fistulae in Crohn's disease. Gut 21: 525–527.
16. Heuman R, Bolin T, Sjödahl R, Tagesson C. 1981. The incidence and course of peri-anal complications and arthralgia after intestinal resection with restoration of continuity for Crohn's disease. Brit J Surg 88: 528–530.
17. Hivet MM, Harmeau H. 1970. Maladie de Crohn colique avec lésions anales et périnéales dominantes. Arch Fr Mal App Dig 59: 481–487.
18. Hobbiss JH, Schofield PF. 1982. Management of peri-anal Crohn's disease. Ann Roy Soc Med 75: 414–417.
19. Homan WP, Tang CK, Thorbjarnarson B. 1976. Anal Lesions Complicating Crohn's Disease. Arch Surg 111: 1333–1335.
20. Kayasseh L, Stalder GA. 1971. Über die analen Komplikationen des Morbus Crohn. Schweiz Med Wschr 101: 760–761.
21. Lockhart Mummery HE. 1985. Anal lesions in Crohn's disease. Br J Surg 77: 95–96.

22. Lockhart Mummery HE. 1975. Crohn's disease: Anal Lesions. Dis Colon Rectum: 200–202.
23. Lockhart Mummery HE. 1965. Pathologic lesions of the anal region associated with Crohn's Disease. Dis Colon Rectum 8: 399–401.
24. Markowitz J, Daum F, Aiges H, Kahn E, Silverberg M, Fisher. 1984. Peri-anal disease in children and adolescents with Crohn's Disease. Gastroenterology 86: 829–33.
25. Marks GG, Ritchie JK, Lockhart Mummery HE. 1981. Anal fistulas in Crohn's Disease. Br J Surg 68: 525–527.
26. Athanasiadis S, Girona J. 1983. Neue Behandlungsmethoden der perianalen Fisteln bei Morbus Crohn. Langenbecks Arch Chir 360: 119–132.
27. Sohn N, Korelitz BI, Weinstein MA. 1980. Ano-rectal Crohn's disease: Definitive surgery for fistulas and recurrent abscesses. Am J Surg 133: 394–397.
28. Lehur PA. 1986. Traitement des lésions anales dans la maladie de Crohn. Gastroenterol Clin Biol 10: 201–203.
29. Mareschal C, Van Heuverzwijn M, Melange M, Fiasse R. 1986. Chirurgie anale dans la maladie de Crohn. Resultats cliniques et fonctionnels. Gastroenterol Clin Biol 10: 204–207.
30. Van Heuverzwijn R, Mayeur S, Fiasse R, Detry R, Dive Ch. 1983. Surgery in anal Crohn's Disease. Coloproctology 5: 105–108.
31. Williams R, Coller JA, Corman M, Nugent C, Malcolm C, Veidenheimer C. 1981. Anal complications in Crohn's Disease. Dis Colon Rectum: 22–24.
32. Slater G, Greenstein A, Aufses AH. 1984. Anal carcinoma in patients with Crohn's disease. Ann Surg 199:348–350.
33. Sommerville KW, Langman MJS, Cruz DJA, Balfour TW, Sully L. 1984. Malignant transformation and anal skin tags in Crohn's disease. Gut 25: 1124–1125.
34. Van Heuverzwijn R, Haot J, Prington J, Detry R, Dive Ch. 1985. Cancer in anal fistulae in Crohn's disease. Coloproctology 7: 23–25.
35. Brandt JL, Bernstein LH, Boley SJ, Frank MS. 1982. Metronidazole therapy for perineal Crohn's disease: a follow-up study. Gastroenterology 83: 383–387.
36. Singleton JW. 1980. Medical therapy of inflammatory bowel disease. Med Clin North Am 64: 1117–1131.
37. Bernstein LH, Frank MS, Brandt LJ, Boley SJ. 1980. Healing of Perineal Crohn's Disease with Metronidazole. Gastroenterology 79: 357–365.
38. Ryan JA. Gracilis muscle flap for the persistent peri-anal sinus of inflammatory bowel disease. Am J Surg 148: 64–70.
39. Keighley MRB, Allan RN. 1985. Dangers of surgical treatment for perianal Crohn's disease. Gut 26: A1136.
40. Buchmann P, Keighley MRB, Allan RN, Thompson H, Alexander-Williams J. 1980. Natural History of Peri-anal Crohn's Disease. Am J Surg 140: 642–644.

3.12 Incontinence after ileo-anal anastomosis

R.J. NICHOLLS

Introduction

Operations aimed to remove the entire large bowel mucosa while avoiding an ileostomy have gone through several modifications since first introduced 40 years ago. The procedure described in 1947 by Ravitch and Sabiston [1] involved a conventional removal of the colon with excision of the mucosa from the rectum leaving a long sleeve of denuded rectal muscle wall. This mucosal proctectomy was then followed by a pull-through procedure in which the small bowel was brought through the rectal sleeve to the anal canal where an ileo-anal anastomosis was performed.

The next major development was the addition of an ileal reservoir into the design by Parks and Nicholls in 1978 [2] with the aim of improving the functional results of the straight ileo-anal anastomosis. Reported results have all shown that this system is superior [3–6].

Since then, there have been various modifications of reservoir design, some of which have been compared by individual surgeons [7, 8]. Some discussion has taken place over the question of avoiding a temporary ileostomy [9] with general opinion being in favour of including this step [10]. The original technique of ileo-anal anastomosis involved leaving a long rectal cuff. It is now clear that this is not necessary, there being no vitiation of function when the gut tube is divided at the level of the ano-rectal junction [8, 11].

While ileostomy avoidance is a laudable aim, this has to be considered as reasonable only provided that the treatment of the disease is adequate and that the functional result is satisfactory. In theory at least, restorative proctocolectomy with ileo-anal anastomosis completely removes all the large bowel mucosa and therefore should fulfill the first requirement. There is now considerable information on function, and indeed the detailed reporting of function after the operation has set new standards for surgeons in assessing their results for any restorative procedure. For example, the operation of colectomy with ileo-rectal anastomosis was never subjected to the same scrutiny of function, neither was low anterior resection.

Continence

The two most important functional variables are frequency of defaecation and continence. Under normal circumstances continence is a function of the anal sphincter mechanism, consistency of stool and the force of expulsion generated in the terminal part of the bowel. In the case of ileo-anal anastomosis, stool consistency is on the whole loose and a natural solid stool does not really occur. Expulsion as represented by the symptom of urgency may be considered to be related to motility of the small bowel. There is evidence [12] that this varies from one individual to another but it may also be related to compliance/capacitance characteristics and possibly to irritability as might occur when there is significant inflammation in the reservoir. Certainly these last two factors are related to frequency of defaecation and urgency is a prominent feature of patients with pouchitis.

It has been known for many years that it is possible to remove the entire rectum and preserve anal function as was shown in patients having colo-anal anastomosis [13]. While there is some reduction in anal canal pressures after ileo-anal anastomosis, anal function is generally preserved although there is only a slight tendency for recovery to occur in time. In patients having ileo-anal anastomosis with and without a pouch, Neale et al. [14] demonstrated a fall in resting anal canal tone from a mean of 85 cm water preoperatively to 50 cm water three months postoperatively. Although this value was not significantly higher at 13 months (56 cm water), Pescatori and Parks [15] reported a modest increase in resting tone in 17 patients having a reservoir operation from 57 cm water at about six months to 67 cm water at a mean interval of 37 months following ileostomy closure. Voluntary contraction pressures in these patients were, however, well within normal limits at both points of follow-up (123 ± 59 cm water, 130 ± 60 cm water respectively), indicating that function of the skeletal musculature of the sphincter mechanism was well preserved.

Clinical results

The starting point when considering continence must be from the clinical results. It is essential to define continence but provided the nature of disturbances of continence are adequately described, it is possible to compare results from different studies. Continence may be normal, i.e. no involuntary loss of faeces, mucus or flatus at any time. There may be incontinence of flatus without other discharge, or there may be a discharge of mucus or faeces. The frequency of such losses should be defined; for example during the day or night, the number of times per week, etc., and it should be stated whether the patient needs a pad for protection. Often patients wear a pad even though leakage is infrequent, for example less than once a week.

Straight versus ileal reservoir reconstruction

There is now considerable evidence that function after ileo-anal anastomosis is superior when a reservoir has been constructed. Heppel et al. [16] showed an inverse relationship between maximal tolerated volume and frequency in patients having a straight ileo-anal anastomosis. Taylor et al. [22] reported a stool frequency of $11 \pm 1/24$ hours compared with $7 \pm 1/24$ hours in patients having straight and reservoir operations. Disturbances in continence occurred in 80% of the former compared with 20% of the latter. Physiological studies of 14 patients after construction of a J pouch versus 11 patients without a reservoir showed no significant difference in anal pressures, maximal tolerated volume or the presence of the rectosphincteric inhibition reflex. However, compliance was significantly greater in patients with an ileal reservoir (9.5 ± 1.3 ml/cm water versus 4.9 ± 0.9 ml/cm water) and the amplitude of pressure waves in the neorectum after feeding was greater in patients with a straight ileo-anal anastomosis. These observations could explain the differences in frequency and continence. Physiological factors which might relate to continence are considered below.

Ileal reservoir

There is now considerable experience of the operation. The continence results from several series are shown in Table 1. It can be seen that soiling is more common at night and if a 24 hour period is considered, faecal soiling occurred in 3%–14% of cases. Completely normal continence both day and night occurred in 29%–76% of patients and minor soiling ranging from 10%–61%.

Table 1. Restorative proctocolectomy with ileal reservoir incontinence (%).

	Day			Night		
	none	minor	faecal	none	minor	faecal
Dozois [3]	75	23	2	48	47	5
Nicholls et al. [4]	75	22	3	75	22	3
Rothenberger et al. [5]	57	39	4	29	61	10
Cohen et al. [17]	n.s.	5	4	n.s.	7	n.s.
Hultén [18]	76		28	48		52
Utsunomiya et al. [20]			7*	76	10	14*

* pouch removed in three patients
n.s. not stated

These figures suggest that there is probably general agreement on the definition of faecal leakage but the considerable variation in the frequency of minor leakage could be accounted for by differing clinical interpretations. The absence of anal leakage should be easy to define yet there is a very wide range of normal continence in these studies.

Clinical factors relating to continence

Continence can be related to the following clinical factors:

Age. In a report of over 300 cases, 75% of patients below the age of 50 years had normal continence compared with 55% of those above 50. There was a corresponding increase in the incidence of 'seepage' in the older age-group (Dozois, 1985). Other series have too few older patients to be able to confirm this observation. Electromyography of the external sphincter in a subgroup of reservoir patients above the age of 40 was abnormal in all cases and abnormalities could be related to impairment of continence [19].

Length of follow-up. Both frequency and continence improve with the passage of time from ileostomy closure. In 17 patients having an S reservoir followed for up to five years, eight (47%) had some disturbance of continence in the first six months but by a mean of three years, only two (12%) were still having difficulties [15].

Complications of the ileo-anal anastomosis. Leakage from the ileo-anal anastomosis may impair subsequent continence, perhaps by leading to fibrosis and some rigidity of the anal sphincter mechanism. Of 50 patients studied in detail by Pescatori and Parks [15], seven had disordered continence. The incidence of stricture formation at the ileo-anal anastomosis was 56% compared with 7% among the 43 patients with normal electromyography (P<0.05). Of interest and perhaps of significance, all patients with disordered continence needed to catheterise while 24 (56%) of the normal group did so.

Original diagnosis. There is firm evidence to show that function is better in patients with a diagnosis of familial adenomatous polyposis compared with ulcerative colitis. Not only frequency but also continence is superior. Dozois [3] reported normal continence in 90% of polyposis patients and in 72% of ulcerative colitis patients. In our own series, 20% of colitics have some disturbance of continence while only 8% with polyposis do so. In Utsunomiya's series [20] of 29 patients of whom 76% had normal continence, the ratio of polyposis to colitic patients was more than 2:1.

Pouchitis. It may be that continence disturbances are related in part to the greater prevalence of inflammation in the reservoir in colitic patients [21]. Pouchitis has only been reported in colitic patients and is characterised by frequency and urgency of defaecation, a watery stool and histopathological signs of severe acute inflammation of reservoir mucosa. The urgency of loose stools may result in soiling. Pouchitis has been reported in 10%–42% of patients [10].

Physiological factors relating to continence

Function of the anal sphincter mechanism

Resting anal canal tone falls postoperatively [14] and seems to remain depressed even up to three years [15]. There has been some debate as to whether results of anal manometry are related to continence. For example, Pescatori and Parks in their study of 50 patients reported resting tone and voluntary contraction pressures in 43 patients with normal continence to be 66 ± 17 cm water and 124 ± 58 cm water compared with 62 ± 20 cm water and 150 ± 23 cm water in the seven patients with continence disturbances [15]. However, Taylor et al. [22], in a physiological study of 25 patients having ileo-anal anastomosis with and without reservoir, resting pressures in those five pouch patients with leakage was 44 cm water compared with 73 ± 6 cm water in the 16 patients with normal continence. In another study there was also a significant difference in resting tone in seven patients with mucous leakage compared with seven patients with normal continence (36.6 ± 9.4 cm water, 78.6 ± 18.6 cm water [23]) although no difference in voluntary contraction pressures was found. The correlation of external sphincter electromyographic abnormalities with disordered continence reported by Stryker et al. [19] is further evidence that sphincter function is an important factor. Only two out of 18 patients with normal electromyograms had continence disturbances compared with seven out of nine with abnormal electromyography. Of 158 patients in the St. Marks's series, two of the eight failures have been due to faecal incontinence. Both had grossly reduced resting and voluntary contraction anal pressures and it was clear that sphincter incompetence was the cause.

The rectosphincteric reflex was reported by Cohen et al. [17] to disappear in all cases, and others have shown a marked reduction in the frequency of it being present, ranging from 5% to 64% of patients in series reported. The significance of this is unknown.

Capacitance and compliance

Capacitance estimations by means of maximal tolerated volume (MTV) measurements using balloon volumemetry have not related to continence. Thus, Taylor et al. [22] and Pescatori and Parks [15] found no difference in MTV values among continent and incontinent patients. However, compliance, certainly in the case of straight ileo-anal anastomosis, may be an important factor. Mean compliance in four straight ileo-anal anastomosis patients with leakage was 4.5 ± 0.5 ml/cm water compared with 9 ± 2 ml/cm water in 16 patients having a straight or reservoir ileo-anal reconstruction with normal continence. In a study comparing three (S), two (J) and four loop (W) reservoirs, compliance in the last group was greatest and was associated with a prevalence of normal continence of 90%, a higher proportion than with the three loop reservoir although compliance was not significantly less. Further work on compliance is necessary.

Motility of the small bowel

Higher amplitude pressure waves in patients with straight ileo-anal anastomosis compared with those with a reservoir have been observed [16]. It is likely that they are related to compliance and they may be the direct means by which frequency is affected. In reservoir patients, gradual filling of the pouch results in the onset of pressure waves lasting 30 seconds and attaining amplitudes of 30–40 mm mercury. This is well above the resting pressure in the empty reservoir of 5–10 mm mercury. The pressure waves are accompanied by an urgency to defaecate and disappear after defaecation. They recur as filling recommences and the interval between defaecation and the return of contractions is related to frequency of defaecation [12]. This interval varies among individuals and may be an important factor in continence. Further work is in progress.

Technical factors possibly related to continence

In the early cases of ileo-anal anastomosis, a long rectal stump was left but this has now been reduced by many surgeons, whereby the bowel is divided at 4–6 cm from the anal verge [10]. There is no clinical evidence that continence has been prejudiced as a result. In the series of S, J and W pouches operated at St. Mark's and St. Thomas's Hospitals, continence has in fact improved in the later cases of J and W reservoirs, despite division of the rectum at about the ano-rectal junction (Table 2).

    The method of rectal dissection whether maintained close to the rectal wall or carried out in the anatomical plain between the rectal mesentery and presacral tissues has not appeared to influence continence (compare Nicholls et al. (1985) and Dozois (1985)) although there is a suggestion that retrograde ejaculation is more common with the latter.

It is possible that the type of reservoir may also affect continence. The only information on this question from a single unit comes from two studies in which reservoir designs were used sequentially (Table 2). The results of Nasmyth et al. (1985) suggest that the latero-lateral reservoir is more prone to continence difficulties and this is supported by Fonkalsrud [24] who reported that 50% of patients had some disturbance. The data with regard to S and J pouches are conflicting. However, both studies in Table 2 report a fairly high rate of minor leakage for S pouches (28%, 55%). The length of follow-up in the St. Mark's series was, however, considerably longer and this might explain the difference. Four loop (W) reservoir function was better than with other reservoir designs. The work of Pescatori and Parks [15] with the S reservoir suggests that either the need for catheterisation or the presence of the distal ileal segment might in some way be responsible for minor leakage. The superiority of the W reservoir which has a similar capacitance and compliance but by lacking the ileal segment avoids catheterisation, supports this. With regard to J and W reservoirs, it is possible that any difference in continence if it truely exists may be partly influenced by improved compliance of the latter. Frequency is significantly improved by the W modification [8] and the normal continence rate of 90% for W reservoirs compared favourably with the results obtained for a large series of J reservoirs reported by Dozois [3].

Table 2. Type of reservoir and continence.

	Triple (S)	Double (J)	Quadruple (W)	Latero-lateral
number	58	12	32	–
Continence				
normal	39 (67)*	9 (75)	29 (91)	
minor leak (pad)	16 (28)	3 (25)	2 (6)	
faecal leak	3 (5)	0	1 (3)	

* () % (Nicholls et al. 1985)

number	9	12	–	4
no leak	4	2		0
>1 minor/week	4	9		4
day	4	8		4
major	0	0		0

(Nasmyth et al. 1986)

Summary

Continence is maintained by physiological factors. After ileo-anal anastomosis, these may be impaired under certain circumstances. The factors include anal sphincter function, compliance/capacitance and small bowel motility. Each may possibly play an independent role although the last two may be linked as, for example, might be postulated to occur in cases of pouch inflammation. Anal sphincter function may be affected by the operation itself, breakdown of the ileo-anal anastomosis, age and the length of follow-up where there is some evidence of a modest improvement in sphincter function with the passage of time. Compliance appears to be important and it is likely that this variable is linked to motility, to the size of reservoir and also to the distensibility of the pouch wall which may be impaired by inflammation as occurs predominently in ulcerative colitis and not polyposis. Motility might also be influenced by the degree of inflammation of the reservoir, but there also appears to be an individual-related factor the nature of which requires further research for elucidation. Compliance and motility are also linked. There is a suggestion that the presence of a distal ileal segment as occurs in the S pouches may be associated with minor leakage, particularly if catheterisation is necessary.

The important question is the practical consequence for the patient. Faecal leakage is uncommon but it would seem reasonable at the present time to conclude that continence will be optimal if: minimal dilatation of the anal sphincter occurs during construction of the ileo-anal anastomosis, that a reservoir of adequate capacity yielding low compliance is used, that there is no complication of the ileo-anal anastomosis and that pouchitis does not occur. Some of these factors are preventable, others are not, and more work is needed to identify risk factors for poor function, not only of incontinence but also of frequency and urgency.

References

1. Ravitch MM, Sabiston DC. 1947. Anal ileostomy with preservation of the sphincter. Surg Gynecol Obstet 84: 1095–1099.
2. Parks AG, Nicholls RJ. 1978. Proctocolectomy without ileostomy for ulcerative colitis. Br Med J 2: 85–88.
3. Dozois RR. 1985. Ileal 'J' pouch-anal anastomosis. Br J Surg 72: Suppl S80–82.
4. Nicholls RJ, Moskowitz RL, Shepherd NA. 1985. Restorative proctocolectomy with ileal reservoir. Br J Surg 72: Suppl S76–79.
5. Rothenberger DA, Wong WD, Buls JG, Goldberg SM. 1985. The S-ileal pouch-anal anastomosis. In: Dozois RR (ed.) Alternatives to conventional ileostomy. Year Book Medical Publishers, Chicago: pp 345–362.

6. Taylor BM, Phillips SF, Kelly KA. 1985. Altered physiology and experimental basis for reservoir. In: Dozois RR (ed.) Alternatives to conventional ileostomy. Year Book Medical Publishers, Chicago: pp 303–318.
7. Nasmyth DG, Williams NS, Johnston D. 1986. Comparison of the function of triplicated and duplicated pelvic ileal reservoirs after mucosal proctectomy and ileo-anal anastomosis for ulcerative colitis and adenomatous polyposis. Br J Surg 73: 361–366.
8. Nicholls RJ, Pezim ME. 1985. Restorative proctocolectomy with ileal reservoir for ulcerative colitis and familial adenomatous polyposis: a comparison of three reservoir designs. Br J Surg 72: 470–472.
9. Thow GB. 1985. Single stage colectomy and mucosal proctectomy with stapled antiperistaltic ileo-anal reservoir. In: Dozois RR (ed.) Alternatives to conventional ileostomy. Year Book Medical Publishers, Chicago: pp 420–432.
10. Symposium 1986. Restorative Proctocolectomy with ileal reservoir. Int J Colorectal Dis 1: 2–19.
11. Beart RW, Metcalf AM, Dozois RR, Kelly KA. 1985. The J ileal pouch-anal anastomosis: the Mayo Clinic experience. In: Dozois RR ed. Alternatives to conventional ileostomy. Year Book Medical Publishers, Chicago: pp 384–401.
12. Stryker SJ, Kelly KA, Phillips SF, Dozois RR, Beart RW. 1986. Anal and neorectal function after ileal pouch-anal anastomosis. Ann Surg 203: 55–61.
13. Lane RHS, Parks AG. 1977. Function of the anal sphincters following colo-anal anastomosis. Br J Surg 64: 596–599.
14. Neale DE, Williams NS, Johnston D. 1982. Rectal, bladder and sexual function after mucosal proctectomy with and without a pelvic ileal reservoir for colitis and polyposis. Br J Surg 69: 599–604.
15. Pescatori M, Parks AG. 1984. The sphincteric and sensory components of preserved continence after ileo-anal reservoir. Surg Gynecol Obstet 158: 517–521.
16. Heppel J, Kelly KA, Phillips SF, Beart RW, Teleander RL, Perrault J. 1982. Physiologic aspects of continence after colectomy, mucosal proctocolectomy and endorectal ileo-anal anastomosis. Ann Surg 195: 435–443.
17. Cohen Z, McLeod RS, Stern H, Grant D, Nordgren S. 1985. The pelvic pouch and ileo-anal anastomosis procedure. Surgical technique and initial results. Am J Surg 150: 601–607.
18. Hultén LF. 1985. The continent ileostomy (Kock's pouch) versus the restorative proctocolectomy (pelvic pouch). World J Surg 9: 952–959.
19. Stryker SJ, Daube JR, Kelly KA, Telander RL, Phillips SF, Beart RW, Dozois RR. 1985. Anal sphincter electromyography after colectomy, mucosal proctectomy and ileo-anal anastomosis. Arch Surg 120: 713–716.
20. Utsunomiya J, Iwama T. 1985. The J ileal pouch-anal anastomosis: the Japanese experience. In: Dozois RR (ed.) Alternatives to conventional ileostomy. Year Book Medical Publishers, Chicago: pp 371–383.
21. Moskowitz RL, Shepherd NA, Nicholls RJ. 1986. Inflammation in the reservoir after restorative proctocolectomy with ileal reservoir. Int J Colorectal Dis (in press).
22. Taylor BM, Cranley B, Kelly KA, Phillips SF, Beart RW, Dozois RR. 1983. A clinicopathological comparison of ileal pouch-anal and straight ileo-anal anastomosis. Ann Surg 198: 462–468.
23. Nicholls RJ, Belleveau P, Neill M, Wilks M, Tabaqchali S. 1981. Restorative proctocolectomy with ileal reservoir: a pathophysiologial assessment. Gut 22: 462–468.
24. Fonkalsrud EW. 1984. Endorectal ileo-anal anastomosis with isoperistaltic ileal reservoir after colectomy and mucosal proctectomy. Ann Surg 199: 151–157.

Index of subjects